St. Anthony's

REENGINEERING THE MEDICAL PRACTICE

Profit Through Efficiency in a Medical Office Environment

Dr. Jon A. Hultman, M.B.A.

St Anthony Publishing

St. Anthony Publishing, Inc.,
11410 Isaac Newton Square
Reston, VA 22090

Limits of Liability and Disclaimer of Warranty

The author and publisher of this book have used their best efforts in preparing the book to provide accurate and current information. This book should not be used as a substitute for competent legal advice regarding any material presented that might be subject to local, state and federal laws and regulations. The author and publisher make no warranty of any kind, expressed or implied, with regard to the material presented within the book.

Technical Editor: Deborah C. Hall, CPC, *director, physician products*

Cover design: Nono Kusuma

Printed in the United States of America

St. Anthony Publishing, Inc., 11410 Isaac Newton Square, Reston VA 22090

ISBN 1-56329-308-0

Reengineering the Medical Practice **"is a relevant, well-thought-out, substantive manual for doctors facing today's competitive medical environment**. It teaches principles of health care economics and operational efficiency in a language understandable to physicians. If you are involved in the delivery of health care today, this book has everything you need in order to survive."

Victor Tabbush, Ph.D., UCLA Graduate School of Management.

"Doctors who don't read [this book] may find themselves in different careers in the near future. Jon Hultman shows how techniques and tools mastered in the corporate arena can help doctors cut costs, maintain quality, and become more efficient by reengineering their practices.

Unlike many books of this genre, Hultman shuns theory and cuts quickly to the chase: which is giving doctors clear, down-to-earth, practical tips they can use instantly. For all those doctors worrying about their ability to survive in a managed-care environment, it provides not simply hope but hard-headed solutions."

Reengineering the Medical Practice "shows how doctors can follow the lead of world-class companies by controlling costs, intensifying their customer focus, and using computers and other technology more efficiently. Loaded with useful, real-life remedies, it shows doctors how to capitalize and profit from the changes that are continuing to change the shape and structure of the medical profession.

The book could do for the business of medicine what *"Reengineering the Corporation"* did for senior managers, namely provide them with a tool-kit for survival."

Randall Poe, The Conference Board

Preface

Let's face it, medicine is a business, and that business is changing fast, very, very fast. The "tried and true" isn't working today, and by tomorrow, it will fail completely. In this more competitive climate, both lower reimbursement rates and higher costs have combined to reduce your profitability and quality of care. To survive, you will need new tools to help you compete profitably and avoid costly mistakes.

The good news is that addressing these problems is not a mysterious proposition. It will, however, require changes in the way you do things. Other industries have experienced similar competitive changes and have adapted successfully. The bad news is that while other industries have adapted successfully, many corporations competing in those industries have failed. This is why *Reengineering the Medical Practice* was written. The same sound business practices that have worked in the corporate arena can be adapted to work in your medical office or clinic. As the practice of medicine and the entire health care industry change, the skills that have worked so well for you in the past must be augmented with business skills designed to improve efficiency and lower costs. This book will provide you with the business knowledge needed to bridge the gap between today's and tomorrow's practice of medicine.

This book was written to teach you efficiency skills necessary for retaining quality and profitability in a discounted-fee environment. Relevant information from each business discipline (operations, marketing, finance, management science, accounting, human resources, economics and statistics) will be introduced where applicable. The concepts presented here can be applied to every medical office and clinic, but those specialties that have high patient volumes and low fees will benefit most from improved efficiency.

In every industry, the most successful firms are those that make the most profit. These profits result from the ability to deliver a high volume of those quality features most valued by the customer in the least costly way. A firm that is unable to deliver a quality product in an efficient manner cannot profit in a competitive market and likely will go out of business. Managed care has the effect of "weeding out" inefficient practitioners from the market of medicine. Glenn Marcus, a Washington, D.C. consultant, has stated that under managed care, "It is not whether you practice bad medicine, but whether your practice style is one that the health plan can or wants to afford." *Reengineering the Medical Practice* was written to prevent you from being one of those practitioners left behind in this confusing new world of managed care.

There are many "easy to learn" cost-reduction strategies. These "easy" strategies will be covered, but other strategies that have a higher cost-reduction potential (such as Continuous Quality Improvement and reengineering methods) will be emphasized. These are not methods that can be learned over a weekend and instituted on Monday morning. This is why some practices will fail.

To understand the difference between types of change, consider a problem that the Ford Motor Company had in the early 1980s. Ford employed more than 500 people in its accounts payable department and realized that it needed to cut costs here in order to better compete against foreign imports. No one was willing to pay more for a Ford simply because of its high cost of paying bills. To accomplish this, Ford planned to install a new computer system with the hope of reducing the head count in accounts payable by 20 percent. Compare this plan to the Mazda company which, during this same time period, employed only five people in its accounts payable department! Mazda's accounts payable process was not simply an improved version of Ford's, it was an entirely different process that had been accomplished through Quality Management and reengineering techniques.

Using comparable logic, insurance plans and managed care organizations are not willing to pay doctors more money simply because those doctors' costs are high. Competing in this new environment requires improved efficiency and productivity. Unfortunately, a change of the magnitude needed cannot be accomplished simply by working harder or "tweaking" the present system. This kind of change requires starting over with a blank piece of paper and redesigning the critical processes within an office or clinic.

This book represents the results of a four-year effort of analyzing and studying other industries that already have been through the same competitive changes that medicine is currently experiencing. All the relevant information needed to compete effectively in a price-competitive market is included in this book, and all the business disciplines needed to understand and implement these concepts in your medical practice or clinic are presented in a language understandable to physicians.

Dr. Jon A. Hultman, M.B.A.

Table of Contents

Preface v

Chapter 1: Understanding the Marketplace 1

The Pendulum 1
Gamesmanship 2
Industry Life Cycles 4
High Quality, Low Cost 7
Introduction to Statistical Methods 9
Creativity and Your Computer 11
Signs of Success 14
A New Environment Needs a New Model 14

Chapter 2: Economics 101: Understanding Relevant Costs for Decision Making 17

Profit Equation 18
Costs and Profit 20
Cost Reduction Versus Revenue Improvement 23
Accounting Costs 25
Opportunity Costs 28
Fixed Costs and Variable Costs 29
Sunk Costs 36
Leverage and Break-Even Analysis 37
Contribution 41
Supply and Demand 42

Chapter 3: Basic Efficiency Concepts 47

History of Probable Science 48
What Is Quality in Medicine? 49
Bottlenecks, Statistical Fluctuations and Hidden Waste 51
Series Lights and the Hidden Bottleneck 51
The Hike: Visible Bottlenecks and Statistical Fluctuations 53
The Freeway and Cycle Time 57
Uncovering Hidden Waste in Your Practice 63
Total Quality Management:
Lower Costs with No Sacrifice in Quality 65

Chapter 4: Basic Analytical Tools 69
Electronic Spreadsheets for Data Analysis 69
Distinguishing the "Vital Few" from the "Trivial Many" 73
Trend Analysis 81
Flowcharts 82
Customer Focus and Cycle Time 85

Chapter 5: Human Resource Development 91
Introduction 91
Employee Cross-training 92
Employee Empowerment: A Few Good People 94
The Funnel Process 96
Implementation of Change 97

Chapter 6: Understanding Processes and Technology 99
What Is a Process? 99
Enabler of Change 100
Computers and Productivity 101
Effective Computer Use 103

Chapter 7: Business Process Improvement and Reengineering 107
Why Process Improvement? 107
Expediting 108
Existing Processes 108
Scope of Change 109
Automation 112
Reengineering 113
Waiting Time, Cycle Time and Customers 115

Chapter 8: Reengineering the Scheduling Process 121
Optimizing the Scheduling Process 123

Chapter 9: Reengineering the Billing Process 131
Data Entry and Billing Process Efficiency 132

Chapter 10: Reengineering the Charting Process 137
Automating Medical Records 138
Cost Benefit 143

Chapter 11: Communication and Work Flow 145
Communication Efficiency 145

Chapter 12: Finance 149

Understanding Pricing Dynamics and Discounted Contracts 149

The Relationships Among Price, Volume and Revenue 151

Discounted Contracts and Profit: A Question of Margins 153

Chapter 13: Managed Care 157

Preparing for Managed Care 157

Provider Selection 159

Understanding Capitation: Part One 160

The Shaller Curve 161

Understanding Capitation: Part Two 164

Where Are Capitation Rates Headed? 171

Chapter 14: Mergers and Acquisitions 175

Mergers and Acquisitions: Optimizing Office Space 175

Chapter 15: The Accounts Payable Process and Accounting 179

Computerized Check Writing for the Accounts Payable Process 179

Chapter 16: Inventory Management 183

Cash Flow and the ABC Inventory Method 183

Epilogue 187

Appendix 1: "Removing Barriers to Organizational Change" 191

Symptoms and Causes of Resistance 191

Diagnosing Resistance 194

Effectively Dealing with Resistance 195

Appendix 2: Trust: A Key to Team Success 199

The Dynamics of Trust 199

Actions Leading to Mistrust 202

Suggestions for Enhancing Team Trust 203

Appendix 3: Medical Office Business Processes 205

Accounts Receivable Management 205

Appointment Management 205

Medical Reporting 205

Human Resource Development 205

Financial Management 206

Inventory Management 206

Patient Flow Management 206

Medical Procedures 206

General Management and Supervision 206

CHAPTER

1

Understanding the Marketplace

The Pendulum

When the "pendulum of change" first swings, it always swings past optimum. This is necessary to gain cooperation and motivate changes in behavior. At first, doctors were unwilling to accept a fee freeze. Now, they are standing in line hoping to receive contracts at significantly reduced fees.

In the case of health care, the pendulum has swung far past optimum. During this transitional period, doctors will have difficulty surviving lower fees. They will need to resist the temptation to reduce quality in order to lower cost. Inefficient medical offices and clinics will have the most difficulty surviving this short-term, transitional period, especially if their patient volume increases during this time.

The downward pressure on fees will continue over the short term. David Chernof, marketing director of Blue Cross, summed this up well when referring to Blue Cross's 6.8 percent fee reduction on Feb. 2, 1995. Chernof stated that, "The fee adjustments reflect what consumers, from individuals to large corporations, are willing to pay for health care. The marketplace is demanding that costs not only be controlled but reduced." Physicians have not yet seen the last of price reductions.

Over the long term, common sense will return to the marketplace in the same way that it has in other industries. The pendulum will ultimately settle back at a point where the highest quality of care can be delivered to the highest number of patients at a competitive price. The primary goal of this book is not simply to teach doctors how to survive the short-term effects of health care reform, but to provide them with the knowledge and skills necessary to streamline and restructure offices or clinics to prosper over the long term.

Gamesmanship

Many doctors are unhappy with the current health care environment, and most of the articles I read cite lower reimbursement rates as the primary reason. I disagree with this conclusion. Instead, I believe that the loss of autonomy and other negative changes accompanying managed care have created an environment where doctors feel helpless and no longer enjoy practicing. If doctors are going to enjoy medicine, I believe the process of adapting to this new environment will have to be more fun.

Business schools compare competition in business to fighting a war. While a good case can be made for this analogy, I prefer to compare it to playing a game. Both games and war involve developing competitive strategies in order to achieve a desired goal, but game playing makes the process of achieving that goal more fun. John Madden, when referring to the salary cap in pro football, said, "When the rules change, the most successful teams are the ones that make the best adjustments." Doctors are being forced to make adjustments to new rules governing a competitive health care system, and while the adjustment process can be difficult, there is no reason it should also be frustrating and depressing.

Many doctors are frustrated and depressed practicing medicine in an environment they don't totally understand, an environment governed by rules that make little sense. Regardless of how stupid the rules seem, or who is to blame for creating them, this type of emotion is counter-productive and distracts "the players" from making appropriate adjustments to the new rules. Unfortunately, even if practitioners recognize the need to learn new skills, they often resent the time and effort required to learn those skills. I believe that the process of learning and using new skills would be more enjoyable if viewed in the context of playing a game.

I still remember the first time I played chess. It was not a lot of fun because I didn't understand the rules and strategy of the game. Each time that I played, it became more enjoyable because I understood the rules and strategy better. While winning was always better than losing, the games were so long that the few seconds of victory were not reward enough to spend time playing the game. Win, lose, or draw, I learned that the process of playing the game also had to be fun. Similarly, if we are to look forward to going to work, the game has to be more fun.

When facing today's competitive medical environment, it makes business sense to approach it as a game. It is also better for your mental health. Remember, it is no fun to play a game when you don't understand the rules or you lack the skills needed to compete effectively. Acquiring skills and developing a coherent strategy is a large part of the fun in playing the game. In medicine, this means "sacrificing" time to attend specialized seminars and classes, reading relevant books and articles (such as *St. Anthony's Reengineering the Medical Practice*), and gathering data for practice analysis. There is no rule saying this endeavor has to be drudgery.

We all have different styles for playing games. We need to know our strengths and weaknesses. While working to improve our weaknesses, we also need to develop a strategy that maximizes our strengths. My strength has always been the ability to develop a strong and diverse offense directed at exploiting my opponent's weaknesses. However, in the early days of managed care, I was uncharacteristically defensive. I was busy protecting turf. There were too many competitors coming after my patients with lower prices. Even though their quality was often lower than mine, it was apparent that price would drive competition more than quality in the short term. Any short-term strategy ignoring that fact would have been unsustainable. It was also apparent that over the long term, when all competitors' prices finally reached the same level, competition would again focus on quality. Playing the game meant surviving the short term while developing a strategy that focused on the long term. This required developing a more difficult strategy that had to include reducing costs as well as increasing quality.

In my experience, I find that the weaker competitors will do the minimum to get by and will copy a strategy that is easy to implement. This usually works well in the short term, but because it is easy to copy, it will not produce a sustainable, competitive advantage. Better strategies require more knowledge, more effort, and are difficult to copy. This is the type of strategy needed to "win" the game. It cannot be done in a day; it will require hard work and a significant investment of time. If it were easy, everyone would do it, and the game would be less fun. The effort, however, will pay off.

How are you going to deploy your pieces (facility, staff, equipment, appointment hours and working capital) in the game of health care? Which will you emphasize more, offense (contracting for more patients) or defense (cutting costs)? Do you understand your opponents' strategies (e.g., rationing of care) well enough to develop one that counteracts them (efficiency and quality improvement)? Do you need to be bigger (mergers) or smaller (downsizing) to improve your position? The game is dynamic. With each movement of a piece, the game board changes and so do the relative strategic positions of the players. This is why playing the game can be fun; no one can retain a superior strategic position indefinitely if competitors are diligent in doing their homework. It is also why you need continuous learning. If you begin viewing strategic analysis and the development of new skills as play, rather than work, it will help you make it through this difficult transition period in health care with your sanity still intact.

Industry Life Cycles

Every industry goes through "life cycle" stages. After a new industry becomes established, it enters a growth period. During this period, industry's market is expanding and there is an increased demand for its services or products. Profit margins are usually high during this period, making it attractive for others to enter the industry. This market can absorb more competitors; it is focused on developing new business and new markets. The skills needed to succeed in this environment are entrepreneurial ones, and the measure of success is revenue (gross income) rather than profit (net income). High fees and steady growth usually offset any negative impact from inefficiencies and higher-than-expected overhead expenses. If profit does decline, the remedy is to raise fees or prices or to provide more services or products.

As an industry matures, the market is no longer expanding, and competition for existing market share (other people's customers) **becomes intense**. A mature market is price sensitive, and there are more sellers than buyers. The skills needed to succeed in this environment are professional management ones, and the measure of success is profit (not revenue). If profit is a problem, the remedy is to become more efficient. **A clear sign of an unsuccessful mature business is one that is increasing in revenue but not in profit.**

The Product Life Cycle graph below demonstrates this concept. At first, there is slow but steady growth. This is followed by a period of accelerated growth that ultimately levels off before a final decline. For each product, service, or industry, the time line of this cycle will be different, but the shape of the curve will be essentially the same. In medicine, the accelerated growth part of the curve (between time points 9 and 17) occurred from the 1960s to the 1980s. The medical marketplace began maturing during the mid-1980s (represented here by time points 17 through 21) and is mature today. The current mature marketplace is on the "flat" portion of the curve and could be located anywhere between time points 21 and 28. Whether the entire industry will decline (beginning near point 29) is unclear. What is clear is that profit will decline for some doctors and increase for others.

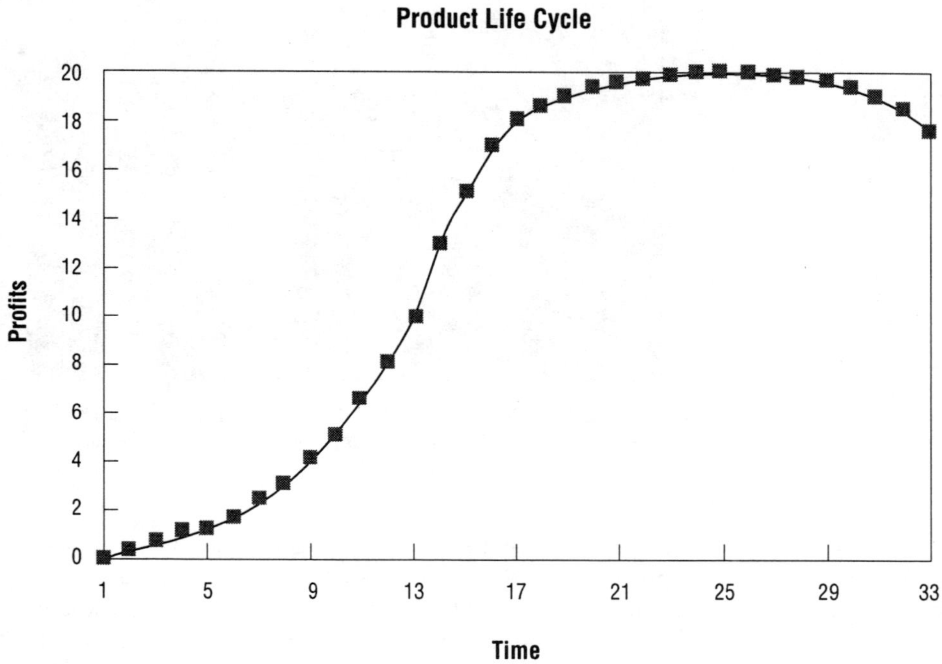

Most doctors possess the strong entrepreneurial skills necessary for a growth market but lack the business skills required for a mature market. The entrepreneurial skills that brought success in the past will not lead to success in the future. This is why so many are now willing to become employed by HMOs. Doctors who will thrive in a highly competitive managed care environment are those who will be able to cut costs and increase efficiency and quality simultaneously. Providing high-quality medical care to the greatest number of people at the lowest price is an "economic good" for society, and it will be rewarded accordingly. This book provides a road map that can lead practitioners step by step to this destination.

While the traditional independent practice of medicine has reached a mature stage, HMOs are still in their growth phase. If you have any doubt of this, you need only observe the profit growth of this industry. I purchased a portfolio of HMO stocks between April 23, 1992, and Sept. 16, 1993. The graph below illustrates the share appreciation of six of those purchases up to Aug. 4, 1994:

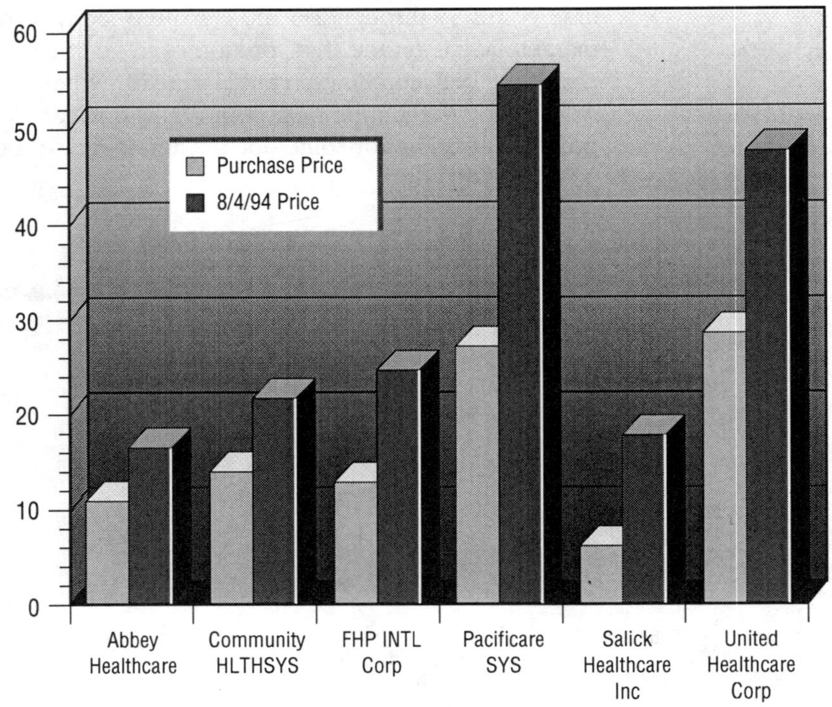

As of August 1994, the poorest performer of this group had appreciated 80 percent, and the top performer had appreciated more than 300 percent. I purchased United Healthcare in May 1993, and it appreciated 100 percent in 16 months. For those who still hope that HMOs and managed care will "go away," the above chart helps to illustrate where Wall Street analysts are placing their bets.

The current condition of HMOs was summed up in the Dec. 21, 1994, issue of *The Wall Street Journal*. The following was its headline: "Money Machines: HMOs Pile Up Billions in Cash as Analysts Wonder What They Will Do with It." My prediction is that HMOs will grow larger and consolidate through mergers and purchases of smaller HMOs. This scenario will reduce the bargaining position of physicians with regard to price.

Following its mature phase, a product life cycle can continue in one of two directions, toward either renewed growth or decline. It took medicine longer than most industries to reach this point because there are formidable entry barriers in this industry. It takes many years of training to become a physician, and specialty training takes the longest. Because of this requisite time investment, medicine also has high exit barriers. The exit barrier is highest for specialty physicians, and this is the area considered by managed care organizations to be in the greatest oversupply. These doctors are not about to give up years of training and quit medicine, but this is precisely what managed care entities feel is necessary in order for managed care to succeed.

When other industries entered their mature phase, inefficient companies were forced to close their doors. The industries became less attractive, resulting in fewer new entrants. This combination of business failures and fewer new entrants ultimately led to price stability. Prices rose from the lowest levels, but they still remained lower than they had been before the mature period. Unlike other industries, medicine still has entrants (new students) entering at the same rate. This can only compound the problem of oversupply.

High Quality, Low Cost

By now, most physicians realize that medical practitioners will continue to face increasing economic pressures. The worst of these pressures is the combination of reduced fees and escalating overhead costs. These same problems have been faced by most other industries as they reached maturity. Each successful industry has initially gone through a period of growth and economic prosperity resulting from high margins. Because of the attractiveness of the industry, others entered and competition began to force prices down. Ultimately, overcapacity and shrinking profit margins forced the weaker competitors out of business.

In the past, a medical practice's growth would automatically "correct" any budgeting or managerial errors. Each year, a practice would generate more income than the prior year, thus "erasing" any management mistakes in financial planning. If practice growth did not fully compensate for poor financial planning, the doctor would "correct" the situation quickly and effortlessly by raising fees, providing additional services, or "enhancing" insurance billing codes.

In the future, success will not come from identifying new procedural codes or practice management "gimmicks" which can be instituted overnight. Rather, it will come from the utilization of superior management techniques which, while not difficult, require time, effort, persistence and the "unlearning" of traditional concepts.

While productivity in manufacturing has been steadily improving as a result of fully implementing such management techniques, the same has not been true in the services sector, despite the fact that the problems and solutions faced by them are the same. For health care, solutions need to be creatively modified and adapted in a manner that improves efficiency and reduces costs without reducing the quality of medical care.

Fortunately, the medical practitioner's strongest price competitors (HMOs) have been slow to implement these newer techniques, but they are now beginning. Knowledgeable private practitioners will be able to reorganize their offices faster than HMOs because their smaller size favors more rapid implementation of new techniques.

Formerly, doctors were taught that there were tradeoffs between cost and quality and that one had to decide to be either low-cost/low-quality or high-cost/high-quality physicians. When foreign products both high in quality and low in cost first entered this country, manufacturers here cried foul because they thought that this was impossible. They have since learned differently!

Cost-cutting by itself usually results in lower quality products that, in turn, result in an inferior competitive position. In the case of health care, lower fees might win a contract, but the delivery of high-quality care will be required to keep that contract. Cost-cutting alone will not "do the trick." The businesses in other industries that have remained successful are those that have been able to adapt quality management and reengineering methods to their specific cost and efficiency problems. They have been able to not only cut costs but also maintain quality, a goal that we in medicine must achieve.

Most HMOs continue to focus on cost reduction at the expense of quality improvement. With this focus, HMOs will respond more slowly to market needs, be less flexible and deliver a lower-quality service. Firms in other industries estimate the "cost of inefficiency" to be at least 15 to 30 percent of revenues. This is a result of the higher overhead and lost revenue due to inefficiencies. Traditionally, the higher margins present in medicine have been able to tolerate a high level of inefficiency. Today, however, a 15 to 30 percent revenue loss can mean the difference between the success or failure of a practice.

Organizational techniques and relevant information necessary to implement efficiency improvements in a medical office or ambulatory health care facility will be presented here. Implementing these should lead to lower costs and higher quality. Medicine will continue to move in the direction of reduced fee contracts. As it does, practitioners utilizing these sound business practices will be in a much stronger position to profitably accept discount contracts and still offer a quality of care superior to that of the competition. If they can do this, they should maintain or improve their position in this new market.

A great deal has been written in business literature discussing these issues as they relate to large organizations. The challenge now is to adapt this knowledge to smaller organizations such as solo medical practices, group medical practices and multispecialty medical clinics.

Introduction to Statistical Methods

Most future changes in the business of medicine will be dominated by data and statistics. Statistical methods are routinely used by actuaries for determining capitation rates, by researchers for defining "good outcomes" and by reviewers for determining appropriate utilization of covered services. In the January 1995 issue of *Kiplinger's Personal Finance Magazine*, Kaiser Permanente employee Sandra Boyd Davis stated, "I was hired because I'm a research analyst, not because I knew anything about health care. This job paid more than any academic position that I could have gotten." The fate of most doctors rests in the hands of just such statisticians and actuaries who have little understanding of health care delivery issues.

A more immediate reason for gaining a better understanding of statistical methods is that many of the efficiency techniques to be discussed in this book require a basic understanding of statistics. While these methods can be complicated, those that are relevant to cost-reduction will be presented in an uncomplicated manner in Chapter 3. It is important to thoroughly understand that chapter because the concepts presented will form the foundation for analysis later in the book and in your practice. Much of this information is based on observations that you have made in "everyday living," but you may not have made the connection between these "statistical events" and the high costs and inefficiencies that develop when managing a medical practice or clinic. You need to learn how to use this information for understanding processes and determining in advance whether your proposed solutions to problems in your practice or clinic will "work" (i.e., lower costs and increase quality).

"Quality control" was traditionally one of the most expensive aspects of U.S. manufacturing. Conventional wisdom held that the highest level of quality could be achieved in manufacturing only if **every** item produced was inspected. This method identified defective items which would then be repaired before reaching the consumer. It has since been determined that this is a high-cost method of quality control because it requires so many quality inspectors. It is also an inferior method because it does nothing to prevent the causes of poor quality.

While the United States was using an "inspect every item" method of quality control, its foreign competitors were using a lower-cost method known as Statistical Process Control. Rather than inspecting every item, a small quantity of a product was randomly sampled. If a defect was found that was outside the limits of statistical tolerance, the entire process was stopped (and not begun again) until the **cause** of the defect was found and fixed. This not only resulted in lowering total costs; it also improved quality.

The primary difference between these two described methods of quality control is that **Statistical Process Control is a preventative rather than a reactive method** (such as inspecting every item produced). One common phrase used by engineers to describe past U.S. manufacturing processes was, "There is never time to do it right, but there is always time to do it over." Doing things right the first time not only saves money, it also produces a consistently higher-quality product and produces it faster. As we will see later, "doing things faster" and "focusing on the customer" define the same statistical concept. In a highly competitive environment, speed provides a significant competitive advantage.

Quality control utilized in the business component of medicine is still of the "inspect every item" mentality. Consider each insurance form that is first inspected by an office staff member and then by the third-party payer's staff. Often, the cost of inspection can be equal to the amount of payment, especially if the inspection results in denials or requests for more information that lead to subsequent "inspection" or further letters by both the doctor and the third-party payer. The cost of this "inspection" process is far greater than the money it saves, and the time spent by the doctor in this process gives him or her less time to spend with patients, ultimately leading to poorer-quality patient care.

The irony is that while statistical methods are not being used in the "business" of health care, they are routinely used by doctors for the actual practice of medicine. For example, consider a routine white blood cell count. This test employs the same sampling method used in Statistical Process Control. A sample of blood is drawn, and from this sample, an estimate of the universe of white blood cells present in the entire body is made. For example, assume that the lab value result for a patient's white blood cell count is 5,600. The white blood cell count is an estimate and has a variance. It could be restated as 5,600 ± 300. There is a 99 percent probability that the "real" white blood cell count is somewhere within the range of 5,300 to 5,900.

If a more accurate measurement (5,600 ± 200) were possible at a higher cost, it would not be worth the additional cost (your first introduction to cost/benefit analysis) because the diagnosis and treatment would not be altered by this insignificant change. On the other hand, if the test gave a range of 5,600 ± 7,900, the estimate would be useless for clinical purposes because the variance would be too large. A more reliable method would have to be developed for the white cell count to be clinically useful. Doctors know what a reasonable goal for this test is. In the same way, statistical methods will assist doctors in determining reasonable goals for improving business procedures within their facilities.

Quality improvement can be monitored statistically by measuring the size of a variance and focusing on ideas for reducing it to an economic minimum. Once a good outcome is defined for each medical procedure or business process, focusing on decreasing the size of variance for that outcome will increase quality by assuring consistency. An optimum variance point is reached when the cost of any additional improvement becomes greater than the benefit that will be achieved from it (here the variance reaches an economic minimum). In the case of a white blood cell count, a 100 percent accurate number can be achieved only by draining all the blood from an individual and then counting every cell. This, obviously, is beyond the optimum point of variance.

While the applicable statistical concepts for cost-reduction and efficiency improvement will be discussed fully in Chapter 3, the white blood cell count example is a good introduction to a subject that will have business applications later in this book. The application of these methods for cost-cutting and efficiency improvement will be limited only by your imagination. Even those who do not think of themselves as creative can improve their creative thinking skills, especially utilizing computers to facilitate the process.

Creativity and Your Computer

There is no one "best" way for doing anything. Similarly, no "best" method exists for competing under managed care. One thing we have learned from other industries is that if we wish to develop better methods for competing, we will need to think creatively. Creative thinking begins with the generation of ideas. Ideas are initially cost-less and risk-less. In a medical facility, ideas should be generated by the entire staff. Later, they need to be passed through a funnel that allows only the few, best ideas to survive. In medicine, the best ideas are those that will provide the greatest benefit to the patient for the lowest cost. Both the generation and testing of ideas can be facilitated by the use of a computer.

Creative thinking begins with raw data, something that your computer contains in abundance. All of us receive similar data and information, but we don't all interpret this data or react to it in the same way. Betty Edwards, author of *Drawing on the Right Side of the Brain*, states that, "A creative person is one who can process in new ways the information directly at hand—the ordinary sensory data available to all of us." For Sir Alexander Fleming, this "ordinary data" came in the form of fungus found on a petri dish. While others had discarded identical petri dishes because fungus had "ruined" their experiments, Fleming's was the spark that led to the discovery of penicillin.

Creative thinking requires the gathering of ordinary data and the "creative" transformation of that data into something new and useful. Computers can be an invaluable tool in this process. Although they cannot "think creatively" or transform data into commercially viable products or services, computers are highly efficient for gathering, storing and retrieving data. While your computer will not generate the creative process, it will be able to facilitate it, and this is a capability worth taking advantage of to the fullest. The software necessary to facilitate the creative thinking needed in your office is probably already in place in your personal computer.

We are all bombarded with raw data from many sources. These data are essential for providing the level of understanding necessary for creative thinking, but most doctors rarely analyze primary data. Instead, they prefer to receive other people's interpretations, analyses and reports derived from these data. Typical examples are the reports received from accountants. While these reports may be useful for filing taxes, they are generally useless for understanding the underlying dynamics of how such things as the number of treatment rooms, number of office employees, variable costs, fixed costs, patient volume and fees affect a particular practice. Let us examine some of the ways that computers might provide the spark that will stimulate your creative thinking.

Database software assists the creative process through the accumulation, storage and organization of data for future retrieval. **The essential tasks that computer databases facilitate are the quick and accurate retrieval and feedback of information**. Speed is essential because a creative thought can vanish quickly.

It has been stated that creativity increases as risk-taking increases. Computers can help build the confidence necessary to take creative leaps by containing the downside of risk. Ideas can be inexpensively tested by building computer models which simulate possible outcomes. Sensitivity testing then can be performed for each outcome by posing "What if?" scenarios using the most current data. Computers allow one to use a greater volume of data and look at more alternatives both faster and more intelligently.

Computer graphics can also help to stimulate creativity. Sometimes data presented in a "visual" format can stimulate a creative idea more effectively than data presented in a written or numerical form. Computer graphics quickly convert numerical data into "visual formats." Pages of numbers may look entirely different when recast in the format of a pie, bar or line graph. Patterns or trends may be noticed that were not as obvious in the numerical form. Also, numbers that are aligned in columns and rows on an electronic spreadsheet may trigger connections leading to a creative thought. It is important that the mind is freed from "crunching numbers" and can, instead, concentrate on the dynamics and relationships among numbers and the degree to which various market forces might affect these relationships.

What electronic spreadsheets are to numbers, word processors are to words. It has been said that the art of writing is rewriting, and word processors facilitate rewriting. A computer frees the mind from the mechanical distractions of writing and editing, making it more open to creative thought.

It should be anticipated that creative thinking will initially create chaos. This occurs because we are being freed from the confines of old models and are opened to the freedom of considering all possibilities, regardless of how impossible they might seem. After chaos has been created, it is necessary to restore order if we are to convert creative new ideas into functional, usable processes. Databases, electronic spreadsheets and word processors have the capability of bringing order out of this chaos.

Once a problem has been analyzed and its underlying causes properly defined, it immediately begins to stimulate "creative thought" directed at solving itself. Remember the adage, "A problem well stated is a problem half solved?" The use of primary data and a computer helps to "state the problem well." The same software used to define the problem then can be used to "test" potential solutions to that problem.

So far, the process of creative thinking has been cost-free. Some solutions require no monetary investment and can be instituted immediately. If a solution requires the purchase of equipment or the employment of more personnel, a computer can assist in determining whether the financial benefit will justify the cost before the money is spent.

Using computers to facilitate creative thinking can be fun. For me, it is much like playing a game in which the data are clues, and the more clues I have, the better are my chances of winning the game. The best way to start "playing this game" is to go to your computer and begin entering raw data. Later chapters in this book will discuss the types of data needed and what to look for during your analysis.

Signs of Success

In the past, "bragging rights" belonged to those doctors who could boast a long waiting time for patients requesting an appointment, a long wait for patients in the reception room, a large number of office employees, high fees and high revenue (gross income). In the future, "bragging rights" will belong to those highly efficient doctors who are able to offer flexible appointing times, have acceptable waiting time in their reception rooms, have an optimum (small) number of employees who work as a team and have low-cost operations that enable them to be profitable in spite of lower reimbursement rates.

A New Environment Needs a New Model

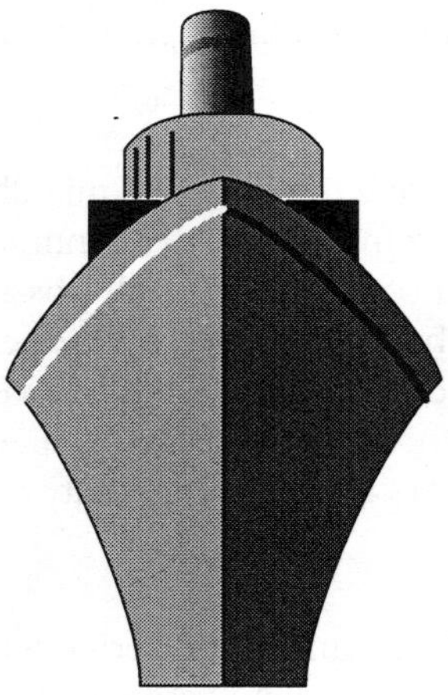

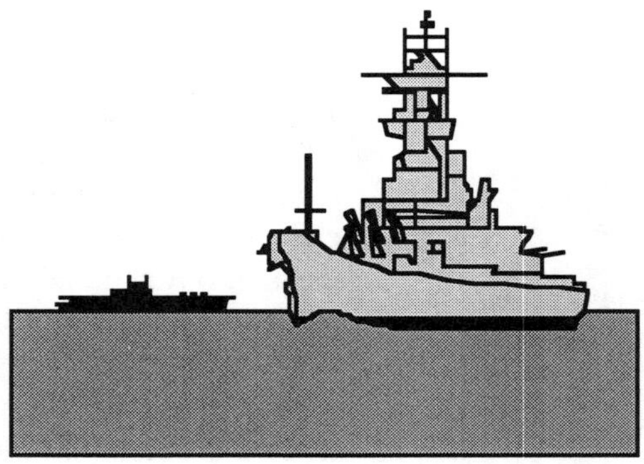

There are different types of business environments, and each requires a different model for optimum performance. The same is true in all businesses. Let us use the ship-building business as an example. Different ships are designed for different environments. One type of ship is not necessarily "better" than another. Rather, each works best in the environment for which it was designed. For example, a luxury liner and a battleship were designed for very different environments. I would prefer a luxury liner for vacationing and a battleship for war. Similarly, there are a variety of medical business models, and each works best in the environment for which it was designed. Most medical practitioners are "fighting the price war" using the "luxury business model," one based on assumptions appropriate for a growth environment and not a mature, price-competitive one.

The business rules that have worked well in the past are not "wrong;" they were based on outdated assumptions and designed for an entirely different environment (a growth market) from today's mature market. Will Rogers stated the problem well when he said that, "It's not what we don't know that gives us trouble, it's what we know that isn't so."

The environment that we are facing today is price-competitive. To succeed in it requires a new set of assumptions and business tools. Remember the adage, "If it isn't broken, don't fix it." Many of us follow this advice, but this philosophy is contrary to the concept of Continuous Quality Improvement and Statistical Process Control. Moshe Rubenstein, a UCLA professor in the School of Engineering and an international lecturer on creative thinking, advises, **"If it isn't broken, break it!" This is the starting point for reengineering**.

Michael Hammer, author of *Reengineering the Corporation*, states, "Most rules and fundamental assumptions that underlie current business operations are obsolete, erroneous, and inappropriate." There are powerful implications for our practices in this statement. Like car manufacturing, medical offices can be viewed as a complex production system. This system includes the transporting of medical records, inventory management, human resource development, accounts payable, insurance billing, accounts receivable management, patient scheduling, medical reporting, patient logistics, medical procedures and many other processes that are driven by a "probable" rather than an "exact" science. Statistical methods can be creatively applied for solving cost and quality issues present in medicine just as successfully as they have been used in manufacturing.

One of the most important habits you can develop is the routine questioning and checking of underlying assumptions on which your arguments are based. Most people will routinely accept the conclusions of a report generated by a computer. Sometimes they will check the numbers. The important things to check, however, are the assumptions on which the numbers and conclusions were based. The numbers will usually "add up," but the underlying assumptions on which they were based are often wrong.

For example, the entire health care reform movement is based on the assumption that health care costs represent too high a percentage of our country's gross national product. I believe this assumption to be incorrect. Consider that as individuals earn more money, their health becomes more important to them, and they are willing to spend a higher percentage of their income on health care. What is true for individuals is also true for nations. The United States is a wealthy nation, and a wealthy nation should be willing to spend a higher percentage of its income on the health care of its citizens. It is erroneous to compare the health care expenditures of the United States to those of nations that are less wealthy.

What if the underlying assumption of the health care reform movement were that there is too much waste (paperwork and bureaucracy) in the system and that the reward structure needs to be realigned with desired outcomes to eliminate the incentive for overutilization and unnecessary care? Correcting these problems would reduce costs and increase quality without dismantling the old delivery system and without redistributing money to "new players" who add no value to the actual delivery of health care.

Most doctors cannot predict whether they will be successful in securing contracts under managed care. If they are successful, they will need to be prepared for more volume, but if they are not, they need to be prepared for less. **Either scenario requires reducing cost and increasing efficiency**.

In spite of the future's uncertainty, the correct strategy for preparing for any possibility is the same. Improvements in efficiency that reduce overhead costs and prepare an office for a lower volume of patients are the same improvements needed to prepare for higher volumes of patients. Using techniques to lower costs will ultimately create opportunities for obtaining managed care contracts that will increase volume. Even if the managed care movement collapses, those who are more efficient will make more profit working fewer hours.

This all means that in spite of future uncertainty, the strategy for survival is the same for everyone (regardless of individual goals). The old business model evolved in a calmer and less competitive market. It will not perform at the level necessary to survive the turbulent cost-competitive environment ahead. This book will provide you with a blueprint for building a new model, one capable of navigating even the most uncertain environment.

CHAPTER

2

Economics 101: Understanding Relevant Costs for Decision Making

The headline on the front cover of the November 1993 issue of *Business Week* read as follows: "STUCK! How Companies Cope When They Can't Raise Prices." Raising prices is a "no thinker" strategy for increasing revenue. If profit is declining for any reason, a fee increase is the fastest and easiest solution. I remember one doctor who, in 1970, wanted to slow down and treat fewer patients. He decided to double his fees. He thought that this would immediately reduce patient volume while keeping his revenue at a constant level. Instead, this action reduced his volume very little and substantially increased his income. The doctor was not able to slow down, but he was making more money for his efforts.

When a fee increase has results like this, when it increases revenue at a higher rate than it decreases volume, the fees are said to be in the **inelastic** range. Fees are usually in the inelastic range in a growth market, and **when fees are inelastic, an increase in fees will increase revenue**.

Few doctors understand the relationship between price and volume, especially as it applies to a health care facility operating in a managed care environment. If profit is declining, as it might in today's more competitive environment, raising fees is not a viable option for increasing profit. In this kind of market, fees are said to be in the **elastic** range. A fee increase will decrease patient volume at a higher rate than it will increase revenue, thus producing even less profit. **The only option for increasing profit in today's mature market is to decrease operating costs or increase patient volume (or both).**

When medical fees first began to decline, most doctors compensated by working harder. This included both treating more patients and providing more services per patient. **Health care expenditures continued to grow under discounted fee-for-service because more services per patient meant more income to doctors.** This failure to control health care expenditures led to the replacement of PPOs by HMOs. HMOs are better able to control health care expenditures by changing the reward system and by reducing the supply of medical and surgical services available (controlling utilization). **Under capitated managed care, more services per patient means more cost for the doctor.** Under a system where prices cannot be increased and the provision of additional services raises a doctor's cost, revenue can be increased only by treating a higher volume of patients. When developing a strategy for this environment, profit, not revenue, becomes the relevant focus.

Profit Equation

Profit is defined as revenue minus cost (Profit = Revenue - Cost), and revenue is determined by both price and volume (Revenue = Price × Volume). If we combine these two equations, Profit = (Price × Volume) - Cost.

$$Profit = (P \times V) - C$$

In a managed care market, price (P) is out of our control and is certain to decrease.

$$Profit = (P\downarrow \times V) - C$$

Volume (V) is also out of our direct control, and it could move in either direction (increase or decrease).

$$Profit = (P\downarrow \times V\downarrow\uparrow) - C$$

Cost is the only part of the equation under our direct control, and it could also move in either direction.

$$Profit = (P\downarrow \times V\downarrow\uparrow) - C\downarrow\uparrow$$

It can be seen from this profit equation that an increase in volume or a decrease in cost, or the combination of both, could offset a decline in profit resulting from lower prices. This is the "winning" strategy.

$$Profit = (P\downarrow \times V\uparrow) - C\downarrow$$

The "survival" strategy will be to decrease cost while maintaining or increasing volume.

$$Profit = (P\downarrow \times V) - C\downarrow\downarrow$$

If volume declines, costs must be reduced to the maximum. Both "winning" and "survival" strategies include reducing costs. **Any strategy that ignores costs is a "losing" one and will result in failure.** While practitioners fear the possibility of failing because of an inability to secure contracts, they may also fail if they increase volume by obtaining contracts that cause costs to increase at a faster rate than revenue. Costs are the key here and they need to be examined closely.

Losing Strategies

$$Profit = (P\downarrow \times V\uparrow) - C\uparrow\uparrow$$

$$Profit = (P\downarrow \times V\downarrow) - C$$

Cost-cutting should not be simply a matter of spending less or "doing without." This type of cost-cutting results in lower quality, especially as volume increases. In order to make dramatic cost reductions, cost and volume need to be considered together. The key to success is to simultaneously decrease cost and increase volume without lowering quality. This strategy is possible because volume, cost and quality are all tied to efficiency. **An efficient facility has a low-cost position and can add volume without increasing fixed cost.** Cutting costs is essential, and improving efficiency allows a facility to reduce the average cost-per-patient by spreading a greater volume of patients over the same fixed costs, thus producing a "relative" rather than an "actual" cost reduction.

Cost cutting cannot be focused entirely on costs because cost and volume are related. Increasing volume tends to raise costs. Returning to the profit equation:

$$Profit = Price \times Volume - Costs$$

$$Profit = (P \times V) - C$$

It can be seen that profit can be increased by increasing volume while holding costs constant or by lowering costs without damaging the operational infrastructure needed to support the same, or greater, volume. **Efficiency addresses both cost and volume simultaneously**.

Costs and Profit

Let us discuss **costs** and their relationship to profit. Controlling costs is the key to increasing profit in the new highly competitive environment of managed care. Understanding the costs relevant for making decisions is essential, and this chapter will give you the basics. It is important to understand the information contained here because a lot of misinformation and bad advice is given by "experts" and accountants regarding costs. The principles are simple to understand, but you will need a new mind-set to understand the difference between "accounting numbers" and "strategic numbers."

Over the lifetime of a business, costs tend to follow a "U"-shaped curve. At first, they decrease rapidly as volume increases. This is an intuitive concept, and most people understand this relationship as being related to cost-savings resulting from "economies of scale." If the annual overhead of an office is $250,000 and only one patient is treated, the total cost of treating that one patient is $250,000. If two patients are treated, the cost is reduced to $125,000 per patient. Adding just one patient cuts costs per patient in half. If 1,000 patients are treated, the cost is $250 per patient. Treating one more patient (patient number 1,001) reduces costs by only $00.25 per patient. As you can see, cost-per-patient continues to decline at this point, but at a much slower rate.

Additional volume helps to reduce cost by spreading the overhead over a greater number of patients. At the beginning of this example, adding just one more patient reduced costs by $125,000; however, adding the 1,001st patient reduced costs by only $00.25. The above example does not account for the amount that costs go up as each patient is added. Each additional patient adds a small incremental cost related to supplies, and when a certain patient volume is reached, additional personnel may be required to deal with the higher volume. At this point, adding volume may raise cost enough to actually lower profit. As patient volume reaches beyond office or clinic capacity, costs rise faster. This phenomenon is related to inefficiencies that occur in a suboptimal environment (such as one with inadequate treatment space or redundant employees).

The example above is depicted in the "U"-shaped cost curve on the following chart:

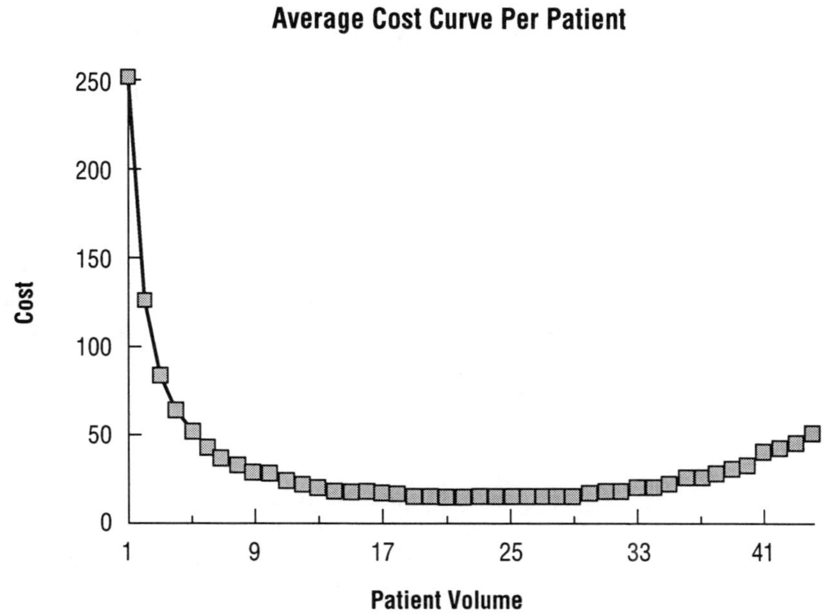

This curve is common to all businesses and shows clearly how the per patient cost initially drops quickly as patient volume increases. An optimum point is eventually reached as per patient costs level off to a minimum (the section of curve in this graph between points 23 and 28). This point is different for each practice and reflects overall office efficiency. To determine the actual number for any particular office, such factors as the number of treatment rooms, type of equipment available, business processes, treatment processes, physician skills and other factors that vary from clinic to clinic must be taken into account. Note that revenue is not a relevant facctor in determining the optimum number of patients to treat; no matter what the total revenue is, profit will be highest at the point on the cost curve where per patient costs are lowest.

Remember that the above graph represents **average** cost per patient. The reason that the speed of the decline of average cost slows and then stops is that, at some point, the small incremental cost increase (marginal or variable cost) for new or additional business begins to "add up." This increase begins long before the average cost per patient begins to increase. The main thing to understand here is that increasing patient volume beyond some point could reduce profit. **There is some point at which more volume does not translate into more profit**. The lower the fee, the sooner this point is reached.

An important connection to make when examining the above graph is to determine where your practice is functioning along this curve. If your clinic is functioning in the inefficient range of the graph (the right side where costs are rising), a volume increase will have a negative impact on profit. This profit problem becomes magnified as volume is increased by means of discount contracting, the addition of new physicians to the practice, or a merger with one or more other practices. Remember that when an office is inefficient, adding volume does not automatically lower cost; worse yet, it can do the opposite. Merging two inefficient facilities can produce one large, inefficient facility.

"*Healthcare Changes—Can Private Practice Survive?*" This is a topic that appeared on a medical conference brochure dated April 1974! It is now more than 20 years later, and private practitioners are still asking the same question. Unfortunately, the changes needed to survive during the past 20 years were relatively simple compared to the changes required for survival today and in the future.

How bad might the future be? Most consultants predict practice revenues will decline by at least 20 percent. While a 20 percent decline may not sound large, if a doctor's overhead is 60 percent, a 20 percent decline translates to a 50 percent reduction in profit! Dr. Lowell Weil of Illinois states, "This means that to capture lost net income, one must either take aggressive steps now to reduce expenses or prepare to increase volume." How does one prepare for a change of this magnitude? I feel that doctors need to do both, and this must be done without lowering the quality of care. The critical word in Dr. Weil's statement is "**now**;" the changes that need to be made will take time.

Dr. Weil gives the option of either increasing patient volume or reducing expenses. Either of these requires improved efficiency in order to succeed. This is true because increasing patient volume has the unpleasant side effect of increasing expenses, and when bidding for contracts, a lower-cost position provides a competitive advantage. Regardless of what ultimate form health care takes, a cost-cutting strategy produces the most opportunities for success and survival.

"Managing the expenditure side of the financial equation is the topic of the decade." This statement appeared in the February 1993 issue of *Trusteeship*. It was directed at college boards of trustees but applies equally well to medical offices and clinics. While we may not always retain complete control of patient volume under managed care, we will always have control over costs. Before proceeding to the next chapter, it will be helpful to understand some basic concepts of cost, especially the difference between increasing profit through revenue improvement (increased revenue) or through cost improvement (reduced cost).

Harry E. Figgie, author of *Cutting Costs*, states that, "There is no more cost-effective way in which a top executive can spend time. Profit improvement through cost reduction is much more beneficial to a company's bottom line than a large increase in sales because it uses less cash and assets. Executives fail to start because few of them know where to start."

Cost Reduction Versus Revenue Improvement

Remember, **our goal is profit improvement**. We have discussed three strategies for profit improvement: 1) increasing revenue; 2) decreasing cost; or 3) a combination of both. It is important to cut costs first. **In a discount fee environment, there is more leverage for increasing profit from cutting costs than from increasing revenue**.

Consider a practice that has $1,000,000 in total revenue and $666,700 in total costs (a 66.67 percent overhead). A 10 percent cost-reduction would equal a **profit** increase of $66,670 (0.10 x $666,700 = $66,670). Assuming a constant overhead percent of 66.67, a 20 percent revenue increase ($200,000) would be another way to achieve a profit increase of $66,670 (.6667 × $200,000 = $133,340 and $200,000 - $133,330 = $66,660). The profit is the same in either scenario, but achieving the revenue increase means that the doctor must manage a substantial number of additional patients.

Practice Change	Revenue	Costs	Profit	% Profit Change
Original	$1,000,000	$666,700	$333,300	
10%Cost ↓	$1,000,000	$600,030	$399,970	+20%
20% Revenue ↑	$1,200,000	$800,040	$399,960	+20%

In this example, either a 10 percent cost-reduction or a 20 percent revenue increase produces the same increase in profit. **With a 33 percent profit margin, cost-reduction provides a leverage of 2 to 1 over a revenue increase!**

Under managed care, it is possible to have a variety of contracts all paying at different rates. As the contracted rate lowers, its contribution to profit (marginal profit) decreases. When faced with a contract decision, it is helpful to compare the projected profit contribution with the lowest percentage cost-reduction needed to provide an equal amount of profit. Again, **the smaller the contract's profit margin, the greater the leverage you have through cost-reduction**.

Consider the same practice in the example above with the decision changed to choosing a contract projected to increase total revenue by 20 percent ($200,000) at a cost of $160,000. The contract's projected profit contribution is $40,000 (a 20 percent profit margin), which will increase total profit by 12 percent. The cost-reduction necessary to increase profit the same amount as this 20 percent revenue increase is only 6 percent. **In this case, a 6 percent cost-reduction is equal to a revenue increase of 20 percent!** With a profit margin of 20 percent, the leverage for cost-cutting is now more than 3 to 1 over a revenue increase.

Practice Change	Revenue	Costs	Profit	% Profit Change
Original	$1,000,000	$666,700	$333,300	
6% Cost ↓	$1,000,000	$626,700	$373,300	+12%
20% Revenue ↑	$1,200,000	$826,700	$373,300	+12%

Profit margins will vary for the same contracts depending on the cost-position and efficiency level of each practice. There are managed care contracts being offered that may provide 5 percent profit margins for some practices.

Practice Change	Revenue	Costs	Profit	% Profit Change
Original	$1,000,000	$666,700	$333,300	
1.5% Cost ↓	$1,000,000	$656,700	$343,300	3%
20% Revenue ↑	$1,200,000	$856,700	$343,300	3%

In this case, a 1.5 percent cost-reduction is equal to a revenue increase of 20 percent. With a profit margin of 5 percent, the leverage for cost-cutting increases to 13 to 1.

From these examples, it can be seen that as the profit margin decreases, the leverage provided by cost-cutting increases. When practitioners are faced with declining incomes, most spend the majority of their time focusing on methods for increasing revenue rather than on reducing costs. This is a carryover from a time when medicine was in a growth market and had high profit margins. In that type of market, it was correct for the primary focus to be placed on revenue and the secondary focus on cost. This has changed.

Even though today's market has changed, most doctors continue to limit their focus to methods directed at producing more revenue. **Most doctors, however, are not suffering from lack of revenue; they are suffering from lack of profit**. Gross practice revenues are far higher than most doctors ever expected to generate when they first opened their offices. Unfortunately, so are their overheads. **In a mature, price-competitive market, the primary emphasis should be on cost-reduction**. The examples above demonstrate the leverage effects of relatively modest cost reductions. Return to the previous examples, and calculate the effects on profit with a 20 percent or 30 percent cost-reduction. This is why reengineering a practice to reduce costs is well worth the time and effort expended.

It is important to focus first on cost-cutting because, if it is done correctly, it not only improves profit but also builds an infrastructure that will open future opportunities for increasing patient volume (and revenue) with less corresponding increase in cost and, thus, higher profit margins.

Accounting Costs

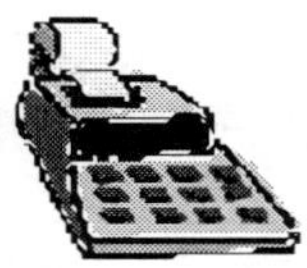

The costs most familiar to doctors are the ones listed under "expenses" on income statements received from accountants. Accounting reports calculate "average costs" and "total costs," but using the costs derived from accounting statements can lead to poor financial decisions. Remember, using wrong assumptions can lead to wrong conclusions.

For example, assume that a clinic spends $20,000 in one year for advertising, and this advertising brings in 100 new patients with a total additional revenue of $30,000 (a net gain of $10,000). The average advertising cost per new patient is $200, and the average revenue per new patient is $300.

Advertising Cost	New Patients	Revenue Per Patient	Total Revenue	Profit
$20,000	100	$300	$30,000	$10,000

Should the clinic make a strategic decision to increase next year's advertising by another $10,000 if it has additional slack time in which to see more patients? This would seem to make sense using the available accounting data; however, the clinic does not have the necessary cost data to make this decision. For example, what if the first $10,000 spent had brought in 80 of the new patients? This means that the second $10,000 brought in only 20. This example demonstrates the law of diminishing marginal returns (each additional dollar spent beyond an optimum point has a decreasing return). The first $10,000 spent on advertising brought in $24,000 in revenue whereas the second $10,000 spent brought in only $6,000. With a loss of $4,000 for the second $10,000, it is clear that this money spent was not cost-effective. This conclusion would not be clear using only total cost and average cost data.

Using typical accounting data, the clinic would make the decision to spend an additional $10,000 on advertising with the expectation of receiving 50 more new patients and $15,000 more in revenue. Using "different" numbers (incremental or marginal numbers), a better financial decision could be made: spend $10,000 **less** on advertising than the previous year. In this case, the year's cost would be $10,000, and the benefit could be predicted to be $24,000 (80 x $300). This decision should result in $14,000 profit instead of $10,000.

Advertising Cost	New Patients	Revenue Per Patient	Total Revenue	Profit
$20,000	100	$300	$30,000	$10,000
$10,000	80	$300	$24,000	$14,000

Compare this with a decision to increase the $20,000 advertising budget by another $10,000 for this next year (a decision that might be made using only average cost and total cost data). This would bring the total advertising cost to $30,000 with a possible benefit of $33,000 (110 x 300). This produces a profit of only $3,000 as compared to $14,000 if the budget is reduced by $10,000 for this next year.

Advertising Cost	New Patients	Revenue Per Patient	Total Revenue	Profit
$20,000	100	$300	$30,000	$10,000
$30,000	110	$300	$33,000	$3,000
$10,000	80	$300	$24,000	$14,000

The reason a clinic would spend money on advertising is to treat a higher volume of patients and thereby increase profits. Today, rather than decisions regarding advertising, doctors will be making decisions of whether or not to accept discount contracts in exchange for receiving a higher volume of patients. In this environment, prices, costs, volume, revenue and profit will behave in a manner similar to the numbers in our advertising budget example. **The goal is to treat the optimum number of patients, not the maximum. This optimum is reached at the point where patient volume, fee-per-patient, and cost-per-patient produce the highest profit, not the highest revenue.**

Most doctors use accountants as their primary source of financial information and advice. Accounting numbers are useful for tax purposes, and they serve as a starting point for evaluating costs; however, if a strategic decision needs to be made (the potential profitability of accepting a contract, the cost of increasing patient volume, or the potential cost savings from computerization), the doctor needs to understand more about the dynamics and relationships among numbers following changes in economic conditions.

Consider the following example: A two-physician clinic's gross revenue last year was $600,000. Total overhead was $360,000 and 6,000 patients were treated. The clinic is offered a contract that will increase patient volume by 1,000 and provide an average payment of $50 per patient. The doctors have adequate slack time available to treat additional patients (an extra two patients each, per day), and they estimate that their supply costs will be $3.00 per patient. Their accountant informs them that they should not accept the contract because their average cost-per-patient last year was $60, and with a $50 payment per patient, they would be losing $10 per patient. This is a common way of thinking, and **this mistake would lose the clinic a potential $47,000 in additional profit** (which would provide a 20 percent increase in each doctor's salary).

	Revenue	Overhead	Patient Volume	Avg. Cost Per Patient	Profit
	A	B	C	B + C	A – B
Old	$600,000	$360,000	6,000	$60.00	$240,000
New	$650,000	$363,000	7,000	$51.86	$287,000

It can be seen from the above table that the "average cost per patient" dropped from $60.00 to $51.86. The $51.86 average cost-per-patient is still higher than the $50 fee received per patient, yet profit, the number we need to emphasize, increased by $47,000! There may be other reasons for not accepting this contract, but the reason should not be lack of profitability. The accountant's mistake is that he was using the wrong "costs" for making a strategic decision. The relevant cost for this decision is the "marginal" cost-per-patient, not the average cost-per-patient (this will be discussed in detail later).

Accounting numbers are used most often for calculations because they are easy to obtain. Two problems with using them are: 1) they are usually based on averages; and 2) they mix both fixed and variable costs together. While this is fine for historical purposes, these numbers are of no value for predicting future cost or revenue changes that might result from strategic decisions that need to be made today. Doctors must know when to use which costs in making decisions.

Two common types of financial decisions doctors will need to become more sophisticated in making a profit in a managed care environment are: 1) predicting how a change in patient volume or fees (up or down) will affect profitability; and 2) predicting which changes to make in business procedures to improve efficiency and lower total costs. The "best" decisions can be made only if the "best" data are used for analyzing problems. For this reason, doctors need to understand relevant costs for making decisions.

Opportunity Costs

There are implied costs to consider when making decisions that do not appear on financial statements. Every time we make a decision, we are choosing between alternatives. There are tradeoffs when choosing one alternative over another. For example, when we choose to schedule a procedure from 8:30 a.m. to 10:30 a.m., we exclude other types of patient care between those hours. Or, if we add space to our business office, we exclude the possibility of using that same space for patient treatment. Decision making requires tradeoffs. One measure of the cost of a decision is the amount of lost profit resulting from that decision, profit that would have been earned had an alternative choice been made. This is referred to as **opportunity cost**, and it can be incurred even when no money is spent. Opportunity cost will not show up on a profit/loss statement, but it should be one of the cost considerations made when forming a decision regarding use of time or capital.

If someone in the office is performing one function, it is always at the exclusion of other possible choices. For example, if a back-office assistant is drawing blood, he or she cannot be changing a dressing or taking an x-ray at the same time. Sometimes, choices involving opportunity costs are made "on the spot," and at other times they are the result of extensive analysis and planning. The latter type of decision is usually more permanent and involves choosing to spend capital or time on one project instead of another. For example, if a doctor decides to enlarge the waiting room, the opportunity to use that space as treatment space is lost.

Opportunity costs are important when making strategic decisions; they are not found in accounting numbers. A dollar-amount can always be put on "the best alternative foregone," and obviously, the use of time should always be for the highest-valued opportunity. (In some cases, a doctor's free time may even be the most valued opportunity.) Opportunity costs become most important when reengineering a practice because many of the decisions made during reengineering involve "who does what and when."

In the early 1970s, "The $100,000 Practice" was a goal to be achieved. I recall a well-known practice management expert stating, "If your practice is generating $100,000 a year, your time is worth $50 an hour. A $50 per hour doctor should not be doing $10 an hour work." This statement does not account for opportunity costs, and taken to the limit, can result in creating support staffs (who do the "less than $50 per hour" work) that are too large and costly and are less efficient than smaller, better-trained staffs.

For example, in the course of a typical day, there may be a few hours when the doctor is producing $400 an hour and other times when he or she is producing nothing. At the times when there are no opportunities to produce income, the doctor's opportunity costs are zero. At such times, the doctor may interrupt an assistant who **is** performing productive work in order to ask him or her to perform a task (a less than $50 per hour one) which the idle doctor could easily perform (i.e., send a fax or book an appointment). If such a need occurs at a time when the doctor's opportunity costs are zero, the doctor is the best person to perform the task at that moment. While these tasks may seem to be relatively "insignificant," failure to consider the doctor's opportunity costs in such "small matters" can result in substantial cost increases and overall inefficiencies.

Fixed Costs and Variable Costs

Two additional types of costs that are essential to understand are **fixed costs and variable costs**. Most data we receive from our accountants give us only average and total costs. Both average and total cost numbers mix fixed and variable costs together. For most of the decisions we will be making (such as short-term pricing and contracting decisions which will alter patient volume), the relevant costs are the variable ones. **Variable costs are the costs that will change as a direct result of implementing a decision**.

Fixed costs, on the other hand, **are costs that are not altered by a decision.** They are a result of previous decisions and are the costs that are not going to change as a result of a new decision. Fixed costs are common to all decisions and should not be a factor in making any decision. Using fixed costs when making short-term, strategic financial decisions leads to poor financial choices, especially when the choice involves a managed care contract that will increase patient volume.

For example: A doctor with a practice grossing $200,000 a year is considering signing a contract that will increase the practice by 2,000 visits a year. The contract will add revenue of $25 per patient and, therefore, should increase revenue by $50,000. Before accepting the contract, the doctor needs to determine the cost of treating these additional patients.

The doctor's accountant analyzes the contract and recommends that it be rejected because, "You will lose money." He explains that the office overhead is 60 percent of total revenues ($120,000) and that the doctor had 4,000 patient visits (80 a week) last year. From these figures, he calculates the average cost-per-patient to be $30.00, and informs the doctor that with the new contract's revenue of only $25 a patient, a loss of $5.00 a patient would result from the contract.

Average cost per patient = $120,000 + 4,000
Average Cost = $30.00

While there may be other reasons for not accepting this contract, anticipated money loss should not be one of them. This type of mistake is made often by otherwise intelligent people. **Fixed costs have been incorrectly accounted for in making this decision**.

Assume that the doctor will be able to add the 2,000 patient visits (eight a day) without any additional cost for more space or hiring additional employees. Furthermore, assume that there is an average $3.00 supply cost for each patient ($6,000 for 2,000 patients). For purposes of this contract decision, rent, salaries, malpractice insurance, automobile, telephone and other expenses should not change. In other words, for purposes of this decision, these are all **fixed expenses**, ones that should not enter into the decision-making process. By using relevant costs (the variable ones only), the doctor determines that this contract will not produce a loss. Instead, it should **increase** profit by $44,000. This is demonstrated in the following table:

(A) Total Revenue	(B) Overhead	(C) Overhead Increase	(D) Total Overhead	(E) Profit	% Profit Increase
			B + C	A – D	
$200,000	$120,000	$0	$120,000	$80,000	0%
$250,000	$120,000	$6,000	$126,000	$124,000	55%

If the doctor determines that treating the additional patients will require adding one more employee, the cost of adding that employee is a variable cost and becomes relevant in making the decision of whether or not to accept the contract. (The amount of this new salary would be added to the "overhead increase" and "total overhead" columns in the chart.)

Confusion is created when some costs traditionally considered to be "fixed" become "variable" because of a change being considered. For example, rent is usually considered a fixed expense when making a decision. However, if a contract is being considered which necessitates that additional space be added to the office in order to manage a significant increase in patient volume, the resultant increase in rent is relevant to the decision being made. The rent increase is added to variable costs at this point. If the current rent is $3,000 a month, and the new rent would be $4,500 a month, the original $3,000 is a fixed expense while the $1,500 increase becomes a variable expense for the purposes of this decision.

Let us consider an everyday example outside of medicine. A simple example is the situation when an out-of-town relative is coming to stay in your guest room for a week. If your house payments are $30,000 a year ($577 a week), utilities are $300 a month ($75 a week), food is $420 a week and extra food will cost $30 a day ($210 a week), what will this guest's one week's stay cost you?

	House Payment	Utilities	Food	Opportunity Cost	Weekly Guest Cost
Fixed Cost	$577	$75	$420	$0	$0
Variable Cost	$0	$0	$210	$0	$210

From these data, an accountant might calculate a cost for one week at $862.

$$\$577 + \$75 + \$210 = \$862$$

However, we intuitively know that it doesn't really cost us that much. In this decision, the rent and utilities are fixed costs and should be irrelevant to making the decision. The only relevant cost in this decision is the variable cost of $210 for food.

What if you normally rent the guest room for $577 a week? This changes the type of decision being made. The guest room is no longer a fixed cost. Having a relative stay in the guest room now loses you the opportunity of earning $577 for rent. This is the **opportunity cost** of having your relative stay, and this lost opportunity is easily quantified. In this example, the cost of having the guest increases from $210 to $787 ($210 + $577).

	House Payment	Utilities	Food	Opportunity Cost	Weekly Guest Cost
Fixed Cost	$577	$75	$420	$0	$0
Variable Cost	$0	$0	$210	$577	$787

Let us consider another example. An airline has a flight from Los Angeles to New York at a price of $400 per passenger. There are 300 seats available on the plane, and 296 are filled. For this flight, the costs are as follows: pilot and nine support personnel, $6,000; gasoline, $15,000; food, $15 per passenger; ground crew, $5,000; and one day's payment on the plane's loan, $12,000. The total cost of the flight is $42,440 ($143.38 per passenger). Four passengers arrive at the last minute and are willing to pay $100 each for the flight.

Cost	Pilot & Crew	Gas	Food	Ground Crew	Plane Loan	Cost per Seat
Fixed	$6,000	$15,000	$4,440	$5,000	$12,000	$143.38
Variable	$0	$0	$60	$0	$0	$15.00

If the airline discounts the rate from $400 to $100 for these four passengers, will it lose or make money?

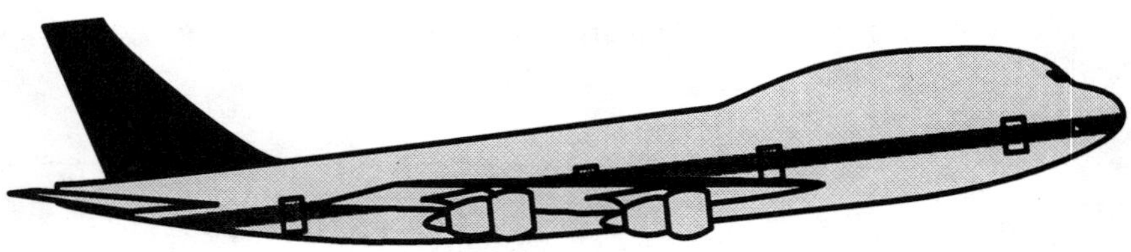

The airline's accountant argues that they will lose $173.52 by discounting the rate for the four passengers.

Accountant's figures:

Revenue = $100 × 4 = $400

Cost = $143.38 × 4 = $573.52

Profit = $400.00 − $573.52 = (−$173.52)

For this decision, however, every cost is fixed except the additional meals. If the food for 300 passengers is already on the plane, even the food cost is fixed. If the airline needs to add four meals, the only cost of adding four more passengers is the variable $60 cost of those meals (4 x $15). The opportunity cost is zero because, at this moment, there is no alternative opportunity to sell the seats for more money. The fixed costs are irrelevant to this decision. The $12,000 loan payment is not only a fixed cost, it is a sunk cost, which we will learn about soon. If the food is already on the plane, the airline will make a profit of $400, rather than lose $173.52, by adding these passengers. Failing to fill the last four seats at a discounted price of $100 each is a $400 profit-opportunity lost to the airline.

We intuitively know that a plane about to take off with four empty seats will not lose money by selling the remaining seats at a discount. This **"discount at the margin"** is profitable, and if the food is already on the plane, increasing the number of passengers from 296 to 300 costs the airline nothing.

What if five passengers, instead of four, show up at the last minute wanting a discount? Increasing from 300 to 301 passengers creates an entirely different situation. To fly one passenger beyond 300 requires commissioning another plane and adding nine more crew members. The decision now becomes, "How many additional passengers are needed, and what should the airline charge each passenger in order to add one more flight and have it be profitable?" In making this decision, almost all the costs that were fixed in the last problem become variable. The airline will not add another flight unless it can cover all costs.

Cost	Pilot & Crew	Gas	Food	Ground Crew	Plane Loan	Cost/Seat
Fixed	$0	$0	$0	$5,000	$12,000	
Variable	$6,000	$15,000	$4,440	$0	$0	$84.80

The total accounting cost for adding this flight is $42,440. However, the $12,000 plane loan portion of this total cost is a "sunk cost" and is not relevant to the decision. The airline will have more incentive to add the flight if there will be some contribution of money to this sunk cost. If it is able to use the same ground crew, that $5,000 cost is fixed. The relevant total cost that the airline must cover to make a profit is $25,440 (the sum of all the variable costs). If all 300 seats of the flight are filled, the break-even ticket cost is $84.80 per seat.

The airline has a pricing dilemma. It needs to cover a minimum variable cost of $25,440 (pilot, crew, gas and food) or cancel the flight. It would like to cover the full cost of $42,440 (which includes the ground crew and plane loan) plus make a profit, but the airline will not cancel the flight if an amount between $25,440 and $42,440 can be generated because this would produce a contribution toward fixed costs (marginal profit for the airline). The airline would like to set an initial ticket price that would cover all costs plus desired profit. The higher the ticket price, the lower the demand will be. If the flight is full, a price of $141.47, or more, per seat will cover all variable and fixed costs. The airline now has to use market data to decide what price above $141.47 will produce the most profit. For example, will they be able to fill the plane at $200 per seat, or will a flight that is three-quarters full at $300 per seat be more profitable? Once the flight is profitable, the airline can consider discounting the remaining seats.

Consider a final scenario: "What if the airline discounts all 300 seats to $80? Rather than discounting at the margin, this is a "discount to the core." Discounting on the margin is always profitable. Discounting to the core would result in a total revenue of $24,000 ($80 x 300). We previously calculated that the total cost of the flight was $42,440. Of that cost, $12,000 was a "sunk" loan payment, and the $5,000 ground crew cost was a fixed cost. In this case, the airline would cancel the flight because, with a total revenue of $24,000, the airline would lose $1,440. It cannot cover its variable costs of $25,440. If the variable cost of providing a service cannot be recovered in revenue, the additional business should be declined. Pricing below variable costs is referred to as "predatory pricing," and it is used occasionally by large companies to gain market share or to drive competitors out of business.

Now, let us relate this airline situation to a medical facility that is considering a discounted contract. All discount contract decisions are similar to the examples above. The key question to ask is, "Does this contract call for a discount at the margin or a discount to the core?" It is essential to make this determination because **the relevant costs will be different depending on the kind of discount with which you are dealing**.

To analyze contract decisions, think of your office as an airplane with some seats empty. The empty seats represent unfilled treatment rooms and openings in your patient schedule. If the contract being considered is a discount at the margin, it is intended to supply you with additional patients that will "fill the empty seats." Your costs for rent, staff, malpractice insurance, equipment and most other expenses are irrelevant for making this decision because they are fixed. The only cost to consider in estimating whether the contract will be profitable is the variable expense of the additional medical supplies needed to treat the new patients that the contract will bring in.

If the contract will supply the clinic with an increase in patient flow large enough to require more employees or another doctor, these new expenses are considered variable and become relevant for purposes of estimating profit. They are added to the supply costs for the new patients. All other expenses are fixed and are irrelevant to the decision. If the contract is so large that it would represent the majority of the practice's patients, all costs are variable for purposes of the decision and must be covered by the contract.

This is not an exact science; however, if you understand the airline example, you will be able to make significantly better financial decisions. **It is essential to determine whether the benefit from a contract will be greater than the costs incurred. Using the correct costs is critical to making that determination**.

Recall the equation: Profit = (Price x Volume) - Cost. From what we now know about costs, we could rewrite this equation as follows: Profit = (Price × Volume) – (Fixed Cost + Variable Cost).

$$Profit = (P \times V) - (FC + VC)$$

This is the equation for total profit, but most contract decisions are based on predicted marginal or additional profit. For these decisions, fixed costs are irrelevant and should not enter into the equation. The profit equation can be rewritten as follows: Marginal Profit = (Price × Volume) – Variable Cost.

$$Marginal\ Profit = (P \times V) - VC$$

It is important to reemphasize that the relevant costs for decision making vary with the type of decision being made. In the above contract and volume examples, variable costs are the relevant costs. We will see later that for cost-cutting and efficiency improvement decisions, fixed-costs are the relevant costs.

PROFIT EQUATION SUMMARY

$Total\ Profit = Revenue - Cost = R - C$

$Revenue = Price \times Volume = P \times V$

$\therefore\ Total\ Profit = (P \times V) - C$

$Total\ Cost = Fixed\ Cost + Variable\ Cost = FC + VC$

$\therefore\ Total\ Profit = (P \times V) - (FC + VC)$

$Marginal\ Profit = (P \times V) - VC$

Sunk Costs

A final cost to consider when making a decision is sunk cost. Sunk cost is similar to fixed costs, but it is a cost that cannot be changed by a decision (even over the long term) and, therefore, should never be a factor in making a strategic decision. For example, assume that you purchase a computer system at a cost of $32,000. Four years later, the system needs to be upgraded at a cost of $16,000. A brand-new system that has the same capabilities as an upgraded old system can be purchased for $9,000. Should the doctor purchase the new system and scrap the old or should he upgrade the old system?

I have seen some very intelligent people choose to upgrade their old systems at a time like this because they argued that they would lose the money already invested. In this case, the $32,000 is a sunk cost and should be considered irrelevant when making the decision. Assuming that the upgrade is essential to the practice, the relevant decision is whether it would be better to spend $9,000 (the new system) or $16,000 (the upgrade) to have a fully functional computer system capable of meeting the office's current demands.

Initially, the answer to the above problem might seem obvious; however, this type of problem can assume many forms, and poor financial decisions are frequently made when questions like this arise. Assume that the money for the $32,000 computer system had been borrowed employing a 10-year bank note at a 9 percent annual interest rate. The payments are $405.36 a month, and there are still six years remaining on the loan payments. Over the next six years the doctor will pay out $29,185.92 ($405.36 x 12 x 6 = $29,185.92). Does this change the decision being made? The loan and the monthly payments are irrelevant to the decision and should not be considered when making it. The loan is a sunk cost; it has to be paid regardless of which decision is made (it is common to both decisions). The loan payments are relevant for cash-flow planning but not for strategic financial decisions.

A final comment on sunk costs: Emotion often enters the picture and confuses the decision-making process. If someone has invested a lot of time or money (usually both) in an idea or a product, it is difficult to "let go" of that idea or product. This is why it can be difficult to sell a losing stock and replace it with a winner. There is plenty of room in clinical medicine for emotion, but emotion has no place in making strategic financial decisions.

If you begin breaking down financial cost decisions into categories which include opportunity cost, fixed cost, variable cost and sunk cost, you will be well on your way to developing an "economic mind-set" rather than an "emotional mind-set." This will make it easier for you to understand the more complicated financial decisions that will be posed later in this book. These include price elasticity, marginal cost, marginal revenue and optimizing cost and revenue. Even at this point, if you thoroughly understand the material already presented, you should have a better understanding for making cost decisions than most CPAs.

Leverage and Break-Even Analysis

In order to create more leverage for increasing profits, there are two important concepts you must know:

- In a price-competitive market, more leverage for increasing profit is gained by reducing costs than by increasing revenue.
- The lower the profit margin, the greater is the leverage created by reducing costs.

In addition to this kind of financial leverage, there is operating leverage to consider. Operating leverage is made possible by efficiencies within the health care facility that make it possible for part of the ongoing costs of business to remain fixed during significant changes in operating volume. Each dollar cut from costs becomes a dollar added to profit, with no resources used up in the process. Increasing revenue, on the other hand, requires an increase in patient volume, which adds costs, thereby giving less return to the bottom line. The treatment of additional patients also requires a greater time commitment from both doctor and staff.

The greatest profit gains will be achieved by focusing on both financial and operational leverage. Both are present in any business, and their respective impact on net profit will tend to be mutually reinforcing. The efficiency changes that will be discussed later are directed at improving both operational and financial leverage. They include a combination of cost-cutting and systems for dealing with patient volume increases. **The key is to be able to increase patient volume with little or no increase in fixed costs.**

To illustrate this concept, the Break-Even Data Table 1 and the Break-Even Graph 1 represent a clinic where the fixed operating costs are $200,000. The average variable cost-per-patient is $22.00. The break-even operations point is reached when the "Revenue" and the "Total Cost" lines intersect—at approximately 2,500 patients. The variable costs ($22.00 x 2,500 = $55,000) plus the fixed costs ($200,000) equal the total costs of $255,000 which, at the break-even point, are equal to the total revenue, resulting in a break-even operation.

Break-Even Data Table 1

Fixed Cost	Var Cost P/P	Rev P/P	Pat Vol	Total Cost	Total Revenue	Net Profit
$200,000	**$22**	**$102**	**2,500**	**$255,000**	**$255,000**	**$0**
$200,000	$22	$102	3,000	$266,000	$306,000	$40,000
$200,000	$22	$102	6,000	$332,000	$612,000	$280,000
$200,000	$22	$102	9,000	$398,000	$918,000	$520,000

Note that variable costs are indicated by the shaded area, allowing the graph to show total costs while distinguishing fixed cost from variable costs.

Break-Even Graph 1

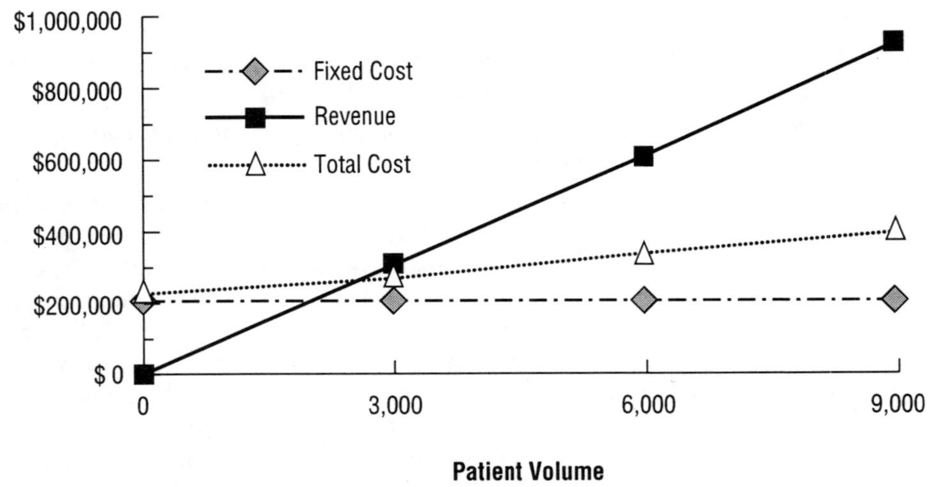

As patient volume increases, it can be seen that total profit (the distance between the "Revenue" line and the "Total Cost" line) increases at a faster rate than does the total cost, indicating significant operating leverage. When patient volume increases from 6,000 to 9,000 (a 50 percent increase), total profit increases from $270,000 to $520,000 (a 92.59 percent increase). **When profit** (not revenue) **is increasing at a faster rate than costs, high operating leverage exists.**

Unfortunately, this leverage also works in reverse. When volume decreases from 9,000 to 6,000 (a 33.33 percent reduction), profit decreases from $520,000 to $270,000 (a 48.08 percent reduction). When volume drops below 3,000, profit drops to zero.

The Break-Even Data Table 1 is based on an average revenue per patient of $102. With managed care's discounted fees, this number will decline. Assume in this example that the average declines to $75.00 per patient (see Break-Even Data Table 2 and Break-Even Graph 2 on the next page). The break-even volume is now approximately 3,774 patients. At this volume, profit is at $22.00 per patient, and at this point, total revenue and total cost are essentially equal. At 6,000 patients, profit is $118,000, and at 9,000 patients, profit is $277,000. To get a "feel" for the leverage effect of a decline in price, assume a price decrease of 26.47 percent (from $102 to $75 per patient). At a patient volume of 9,000, profit would decline by 46.73 percent, and at a patient volume of 6,000, profit would decline by 77.31 percent. How could a multi-doctor office survive such a price reduction?

Break-Even Data Table 2

Fixed Cost	Var Cost P/P	Rev P/P	Pat Vol	Total Cost	Total Revenue	Net Profit
$200,000	$22	$75	2,500	$255,000	$187,500	($67,500)
$200,000	$22	$75	3,000	$266,000	$225,000	($41,000)
$200,000	$22	$75	3,774	$283,028	$283,050	$22
$200,000	$22	$75	6,000	$332,000	$450,000	$118,000
$200,000	$22	$75	9,000	$398,000	$675,000	$277,000

Break-Even Graph 2

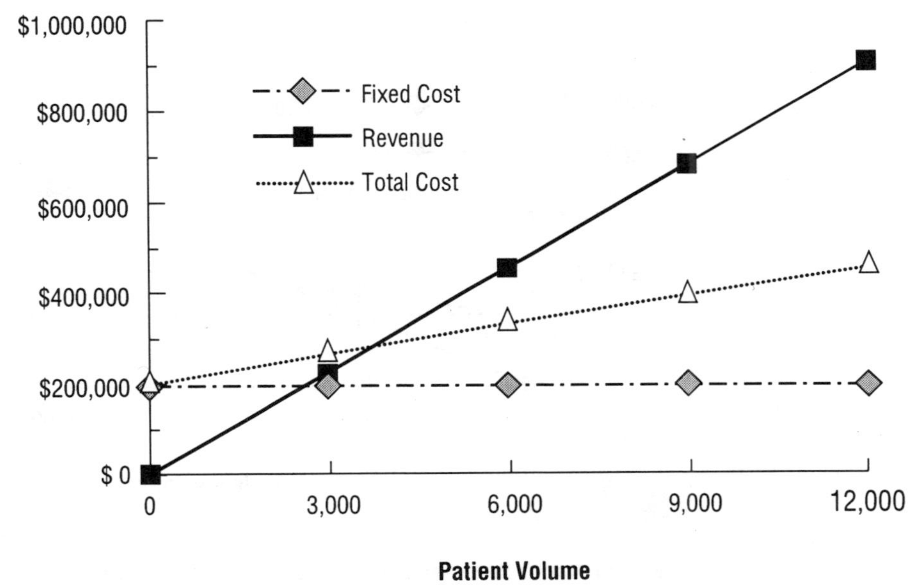

The final scenario to consider is the one most likely to occur under managed care contracting: A decrease in fees, combined with an increase in fixed costs, caused by an increase in both patient volume and the amount and complexity of paperwork required by the managed care organizations.

The Break-Even Table 3 and Break-Even Graph 3 demonstrate the effect on profit caused by an increase in fixed costs from $200,000 to $250,000, combined with a decrease in average revenue per patient of $27.00 (from $102 to $75.00). At a patient volume of 9,000, profit declines by 56 percent. For each of the three doctors, salary would drop from $173,333 to $75,666. If volume dropped to 6,000 patients, profit would decline 87 percent. In order to produce the original profit of $520,000, volume would have to be increased by 61 percent (to 14,528 patients). It is likely that an increase of that magnitude would raise fixed costs substantially and might offset much of the gain in revenue.

Break-Even Data Table 3

Fixed Cost	Var Cost P/P	Rev P/P	Pat Vol	Total Cost	Total Revenue	Net Profit
$250,000	$22	$75	2,500	$305,000	$187,500	($67,500)
$250,000	$22	$75	3,000	$316,000	$225,000	($41,000)
$250,000	$22	$75	4,717	$353,774	$353,775	$1
$250,000	$22	$75	6,000	$382,000	$450,000	$68,000
$250,000	$22	$75	9,000	$448,000	$675,000	$227,000

Break-Even Graph 3

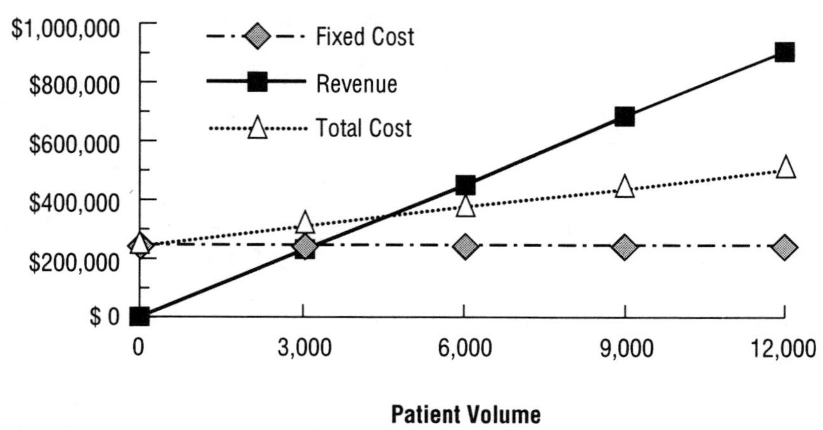

Rather than attempting to increase patient volume by 61 percent, this medical group should consider an aggressive cost-cutting (efficiency improvement) strategy, coupled with a more modest patient volume increase. At a volume of 9,000 patients, cutting fixed and variable costs by 32 percent, as depicted in the next graph, would produce a net profit of $370,000, which represents a 63 percent increase in profit ($123,333 for each doctor). Following this cost-cutting, a volume increase of 20 percent (from 9,000 to 10,781 patients) would be required to achieve the previous net profit of $520,000. This volume increase is more achievable than a 61 percent volume increase, and if the doctors are not able to attain a 20 percent increase in patient volume, they will still "survive" better with the cost reduction. Cutting costs this aggressively requires efficiency changes possible only through quality management and reengineering techniques.

32 Percent Cost Reduction Graph

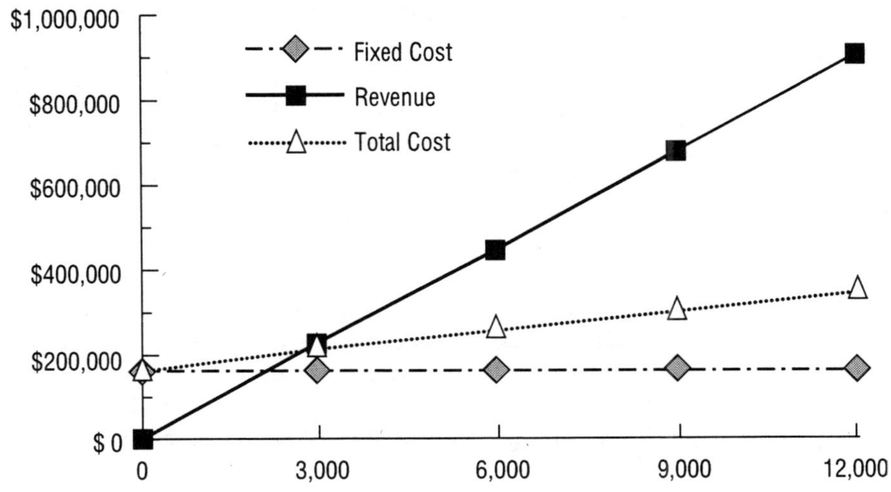

The relationships depicted in the tables and graphs used throughout this book should be reviewed and examined carefully. Relationships among various factors are easier to predict when you are familiar with the "visual" graphs. The graphs demonstrate clearly which variables change in response to others. The **relative magnitude** and **direction** of these changes are also clear. It doesn't matter that exact numbers always be calculated. With this understanding, you will be able to develop a better strategy for any potential change. More importantly, given the type of change predicted for medicine, you will develop a better strategy by knowing which alternatives will provide the greatest leverage.

Contribution

Another concept that can be learned from the previous break-even charts is that of **contribution**. Every service we provide will not always generate enough revenue to cover full costs (fixed cost plus variable cost). **As long as the revenue received from a service is above the variable cost of providing that service, it is said to be making a contribution to the fixed cost**.

In a highly competitive industry, it is common for a business to lower prices in order to gain market share. A business can "afford" to lower prices temporarily as long as it is charging enough to cover an amount greater than its variable costs and is, thereby, making a contribution to fixed costs. The tactic of charging a price below variable costs in order to gain market share is the kind of predatory pricing we saw in the earlier airline example. Obviously, this can be a problem for competitors because, if a business has deep pockets and is able to lower its price below its variable costs for a long enough period of time, it can force its competitors out of business. This lessens competition, and prices will ultimately go up.

If a contract's predicted revenue is above variable costs but does not cover all fixed costs, it should still be considered as long as it provides additional patients and the doctor has the time and the space to treat the patients without adding personnel. Such a contract will add to total profit. **Any contract that is below a practice's variable costs lowers its profit and should never be considered**.

Some doctors, however, are being driven by the "fear of exclusion" from managed care contracting and are entering into contracts that are close to fee structures which are below the variable cost of providing services. While a colleague with lower costs may be in a position to profit from such a contract, it will be of no benefit to you if your cost position is too high.

Supply and Demand

The "law of supply and demand" operates in every market where there are buyers and sellers. Some argue that the medical marketplace is not a "normal" free market and, therefore, does not follow the law of supply and demand. However, the law of supply and demand is useful in predicting how doctors, patients, employers and third-party payers will behave in the medical marketplace in response to price and volume changes.

Price is what stabilizes supply and demand in a market. Aside from natural disasters, "shortages" generally do not exist. If there is a shortage, it usually means that price is too low. If there is a surplus, price is too high. If there are artificial constraints (e.g. rent control, crop subsidies) on the free movement of price, shortages or surpluses develop.

During the "gas shortage" in the mid-1970s, economists could easily predict what the price of gas needed to be in order to end the shortage and eliminate the long lines at gas stations. Some argued that the shortage was related to declining oil reserves; however, when the price reached the magic number (predicted in advance by economists), the "shortage" ended. The price was high enough to "encourage" people to drive less, join car pools, combine errands and, ultimately, to purchase cars that were more fuel-efficient.

When there is a shortage, upward price movement reduces demand, and the "shortage" disappears. If upward price movement shows little effect on demand, sellers begin to supply more of a product or service and take in the profit that is created by higher prices. These "sellers" are willing to work harder in order to supply more, and the business becomes an attractive one for others to enter. As supply is increased by both higher production and more people entering the business, competition and excess supply ultimately push prices down.

So far, medicine has fit this model. As doctors increased prices in medicine, there was little effect on demand because most of the cost was absorbed by third parties, the insurance companies and employers. Doctors were able to increase demand for their services using new technology and procedures. Profit margins were high, and the "best and brightest" wanted to be doctors. High profit margin is obviously not the only reason that people entered medicine, but it has been one of the contributing factors to the current surplus of doctors and hospitals.

Under managed care, there has been an increasing demand from patients for health care services because patients pay less out-of-pocket expenses. Managed care entities, however, are effectively reducing the supply of many services (especially more expensive ones) by paying less for them and placing access barriers to these procedures.

Understanding market response to changes in supply, demand and price is vital in a constantly changing, highly competitive market. Understanding market response is essential in determining all of the following: how patient volume will change in response to fee changes, the effect that deductibles and copayments will have on patient utilization, how noncovered services should be priced and which long-term competitive strategies should be adopted.

The Demand Curve

The demand curve is always downward-sloping. As price declines, the demand for more product or service increases. Graph One: The Demand Curve depicts an example where, at a price of $60.00 for "service or products," there is demand for 1,000 units of that product or service. When the price is reduced to $40.00, the demand increases to 500,000 units. One could reverse this statement and say that if there was a supply (or oversupply) of 500,000 units, the price would have to be set at $40 to sell all of the available units. There is now less incentive for the providers of that product or service to increase supply. As supply declines, prices will stabilize or begin to move upward.

Graph One: The Demand Curve

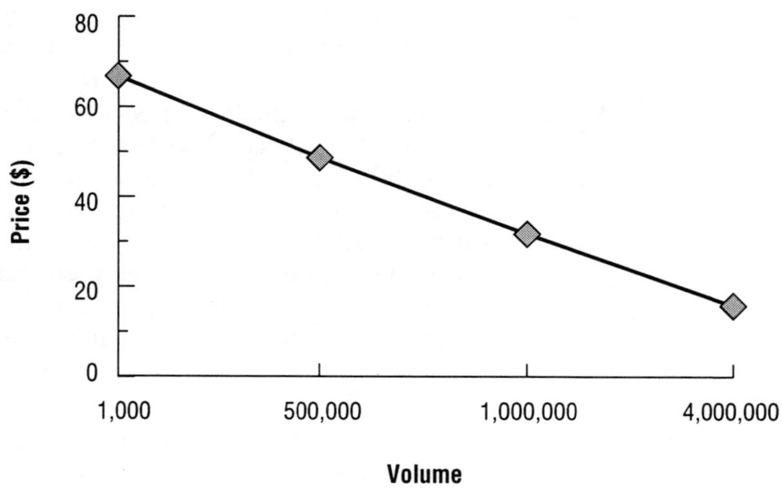

The Supply Curve

The supply curve is always upward-sloping. The higher the price, the greater incentive providers have for supplying more product or service, and the greater incentive there is for other providers to enter the market.

Graph Two: The Supply Curve demonstrates the upward-sloping supply curve. As price is increased, there is a stronger incentive for suppliers to provide more products or services. For the product or service represented by this graph, 500,000 units of the product or service will be supplied at a price of $35. One million units will be supplied at a price of $50. There may not, however, be a market for so great a volume of this product or service at that price.

Graph Two: The Supply Curve

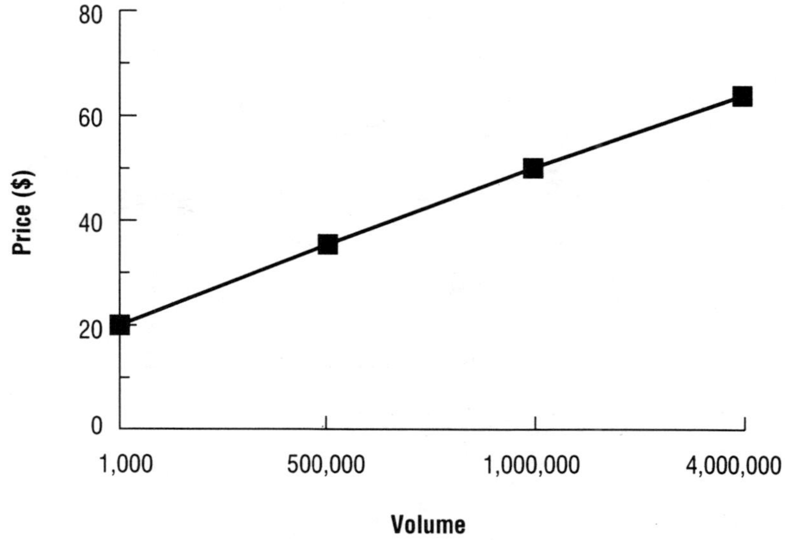

A market is in equilibrium at the point where the supply and demand curves intersect. At this point, there is an equal number of buyers and sellers. This is the point of intersection of the two lines in Graph Three: Supply and Demand Curve on the next page. On this graph, this point occurs at a price of $38.00 and a volume of approximately 600,000 units.

If, in this example, demand increased to 1,000,000 units, an upward pressure would theoretically be placed on price, which would increase to $50.00. If the price remained at $38.00 when the demand increased to 1,000,000, there would be a "shortage" of product or service. This shortage would be eliminated by increasing the price to the optimum market price. Conversely, if the providers overestimated demand and raised the price to $60.00, there would be less demand, and a surplus would develop, putting a downward pressure on price.

Graph Three: Supply and Demand Curve

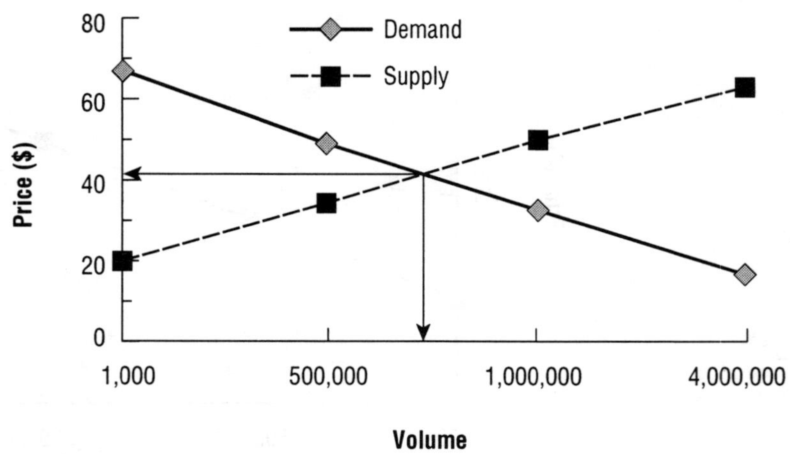

Market forces are constantly shifting as the number of buyers or sellers changes or as consumer preferences change. Every time there is a change in any one of the variables, there is a corresponding change in the others. Again, this is not an exact science, but by using these concepts you will know how to predict the degree and direction of change. The more data you have, the more accurate your estimate will be.

More complex movements of price, volume, cost and elasticity will be discussed in Chapter 12. Understanding these issues will be critical when making contracting decisions requiring reasonably accurate predictions of cost and volume changes.

CHAPTER

3

Basic Efficiency Concepts

Doctors understand the importance of learning basic science for the practice of medicine. Diagnostic and treatment procedures constantly change. Many treatment procedures learned in medical school 20 years ago might even be considered malpractice today! Understanding basic science allows a doctor to develop and evaluate new diagnostic and treatment procedures.

The concepts of basic science remain the same in spite of a constantly changing environment. What is true for diagnostic and treatment procedures is equally true for business processes. The underlying concepts for understanding business procedures, like the laws of science, remain constant. It is important to keep these concepts in mind as you adapt your business procedures to the constantly changing medical marketplace.

These basics will be discussed in the next few chapters and apply equally well to both medical and business processes. While it is important that physicians learn to apply these concepts to both, we will focus on the business processes. Medical processes are under the direct supervision and view of the physician during regular business hours and, for this reason, are easier for the doctor to understand and change. Because of this, they are usually of higher quality too. Doctors are trained to understand medical processes, not business processes. Also, business processes are "out of sight" during normal business hours, the doctor is usually unaware of them, and because of this, they are more difficult to supervise and change.

The high cost of office overhead is due in large part to inefficiencies resulting from poor business processes. **"Fixing" these inefficient business processes is the most important thing you can do to lower costs and improve overall office efficiency.** You will also improve your competitive advantage if you focus on changes that improve the business processes which deliver the services most valued by your "customers." Industrial statisticians have discovered that defects in performance are usually built directly into work processes. Knowledge of the customers' needs and expectations, stated in explicit, measurable terms, is essential for designing processes that can satisfy these customers.

The only "customers" that doctors had to please in the past were patients and referring physicians. Under managed care, however, this list of customers should be expanded to include employers, managed care organizations and regulators. These customers interface with both the doctor and the doctor's business processes. Many of the processes are out of the physician's view but are not beyond his or her control.

One of the goals of this book is to help you achieve quality improvement along with cost-reduction. To do this, you will need to learn scientific and managerial techniques that emphasize system analysis and process improvement. This will require a multidisciplinary approach that draws on systems engineering, organizational development and applied statistics.

History of Probable Science

The concept of interchangeable parts was introduced in the year 1787. At one time, the manufacturing of parts was believed to be an exact science. By 1870 it became clear that no two parts could be made exactly alike; only the degree of variation among parts could be improved. It was determined that even if it were theoretically possible to make parts exactly alike, it would be too costly. This gave birth to probable science, a science that includes statistical concepts, including probability.

Statistical methods help to minimize confusion in the presence of variation. We will learn how to use statistical methods to understand processes, to bring them under control, and finally, to improve them. Statistical knowledge helps in minimizing the cost of inspection required to give adequate assurance of quality; it reduces variability in quality to an **economic minimum**. In health care, the inspection approach takes the form of utilization management. Inspection is the most costly method for quality control, and quality experts unanimously agree that the more inspectors you have, the poorer the quality by definition.

Walter A. Shewart, an AT&T Bell Laboratories physicist, adapted statistical concepts that originated in agricultural research to manufacturing processes. W. Edwards Deming and J.M. Juran, two "quality gurus" who influenced the thinking of Japanese manufacturers in the early 1950s, were both influenced by Walter A. Shewart. Deming introduced Statistical Quality Control to Japanese companies while Juran taught Total Quality Management. Statistical Quality Control replaced the more costly inspection method in Japan and gave the Japanese a competitive advantage over U.S. companies that were slow to change.

Philip Crosby, author of *Quality is Free*, is another "quality guru" who has effectively communicated statistical quality concepts to business people in the United States. It is interesting to note that his early training was in podiatric medicine, and this was one factor that led him to a concept well known to doctors: It is less costly, and better for the patient, to prevent a disease than to treat it. **Prevention of problems is the foundation of cost-reduction and quality improvement**.

While physicians understand such a principle when it is applied in a clinical setting, they seem to have a block when it comes to applying that same principle to operational and financial problems.

What Is Quality in Medicine?

Quality is constantly mentioned as one of the goals of managed care, but few physicians understand what quality means when third-party payers apply the term to medicine. Some physicians argue that, because they provide a higher quality of care than other doctors, they should be paid more money for that care; however, they are unable to demonstrate what differentiates their care and why it should be worth more. John M. Burns, former vice president and medical director for Honeywell, Inc., summed up what large purchasers of health care products believe quality is, "Quality in health care should be defined in the same way that all services and products are acquired, on the basis of the specifications of the purchaser."

When higher-quality cars began arriving in the United States from Japan, people could "see" the difference. The quality of a service is less definable than quality of a product and is often difficult to "see" in medicine. In highly competitive businesses, quality is defined by the customer. The same will be true for medicine. This means that, under managed care, quality will be defined by all of the following customers: patients, employers, government and other third-party payers.

At one time, quality meant the absence of defects. In today's more competitive markets, quality has become the basis of competition and means more than that. In the 1991 book *Quality or Else*, authors Lloyd Dobyns and Clare Crawford-Mason defined quality as "... a better way of producing goods and services, a way that eliminates waste, gives employees pride in their work, and keeps the customer coming back for more. As you produce quality, productivity automatically goes up and costs automatically go down." This definition is one that is equally useful in the delivery of health care, especially since we compete for patients on the basis of both price and quality.

Good outcomes are what doctors and patients perceive as quality, and this is not in conflict with a statistical measure of quality. Once a desired outcome is agreed upon by the majority of doctors, it can be quantified in terms of how consistently, and at what price, that outcome is achieved. The fact that a procedure is performed by a "world-renowned surgeon at a world-class hospital" is irrelevant if the same outcome is achieved at a lower cost by a "lesser-known" doctor at a competing institution.

Deming saw uniformity as one important ingredient of quality. Crosby agreed, and he defined quality as, "conformance to requirements, not goodness, and it is measured by the price of nonconformance." In medicine, the "requirements" need to be defined first and then agreed upon by the majority of physicians. Quality means providing those "requirements" consistently (less variance) and with the least amount of waste. Quality, customer focus and cost-reduction are all compatible and interrelated concepts.

The term "customer focus" is often used when defining quality. Deming is correct when he states that in a competitive market, quality should be considered from the point of view of the user (customer). In the case of managed care, both the patient and the managed care organization are customers. Doctors think that customer focus means only that they should care about their patients and render the best level of care they are capable of delivering. This, however, is **expected** doctor behavior. Quality care and customer focus go beyond this.

Any doctor who signs a managed care contract is expected to be well trained and render compassionate, "high-quality" care. This is the entry level necessary to "play the game." Customer focus in medicine does not refer to these expected, entry-level qualities. It can be measured statistically as **cycle time** (the total time a patient spends in the treatment facility). Doctors who are able to reduce cycle time will be supplying the most efficient care, the kind of high-quality and cost-effective care that is valued by the patient. Before learning about cycle time and how to reduce it, one must first understand how statistical fluctuations, bottlenecks and wasted activities combine to create poor quality and high costs by increasing cycle time. This will make it easier to understand how correcting these problems will lead to the desired goal of higher quality and lower costs.

Bottlenecks, Statistical Fluctuations and Hidden Waste

Bottlenecks, statistical fluctuations and hidden waste affect your practice negatively, and it is essential to understand how to use reengineering techniques to make dramatic improvements in cost, quality and productivity. We will use relatively "simple" examples to explain complicated statistical concepts that affect every area of your practice. I will refer to these examples again when discussing reengineering. It is amazing how many applications these concepts have and the important contributions they can make in helping you analyze and solve problems.

Series Lights and the Hidden Bottleneck

I still remember my first childhood encounter with a set of decorative holiday lights. I had difficulty understanding why one entire strand of bulbs wouldn't light when they were plugged in. When I asked my parents why, they explained that some of the strands were series rather than parallel lights. I discovered that if one bulb in a series strand didn't work, none of the remaining lights would work. On the other hand, if one bulb did not work in a parallel strand, the remaining bulbs would light, making it obvious which one to replace. I wondered why anyone would buy series lights. The answer my parents gave was that they were cheaper, presumably because they were easier to produce.

Just think of the advantage parallel lights had over series lights! In a series strand, one bulb could control all the others. If the strand didn't light, and it contained 100 bulbs, finding the burned-out bulb would require a tedious trial-and-error process. If more than one bulb burned out, it would become almost impossible to find the defective ones without replacing all 100 bulbs with new ones. If this strand of bulbs was used to represent a business, each bulb would have the potential of controlling the quality and productivity of the entire business and, thereby, the profit too.

Even as a child, it seemed to me that the small cost savings of the series lights did not offset the frustration of their not working when they were needed. The cost in time and aggravation of finding the burned-out bulb seemed greater than the initial price differential of the two types of strands. More importantly, if the lights didn't work when they were needed, they were worthless. In this sense, the series lights were actually more costly.

Without realizing it, we have constructed many of our office business processes as dependent series of events similar to the strands of series light bulbs. The slowest activity step in each process (the bottleneck) "limits" the efficiency of that entire process, and that bottleneck step can be as difficult to find as it was to locate a burned-out bulb on a series strand of lights.

Two important concepts are illustrated by the shortcomings of series lights. These concepts can help to explain why it is difficult to find and fix problems that make our business processes less efficient and more costly than they should be.

The first critical concept is that **"fixing" any activity in a dependent series other than the bottleneck adds cost but does not improve the process as a whole**. Fixing a non-bottleneck step is no different than replacing one of the series bulbs that is functional but does not appear to be so because another bulb has failed. It is easy to see that any time or money spent replacing these "working" bulbs improves nothing but adds cost.

The second significant concept is that **a bottleneck can be improved by "paralleling" around it, and this will always improve the entire process.** As we will see later, the concept of "paralleling" around a problem has powerful applications to many of our current business process cost and efficiency problems. More importantly, if a process is constructed in parallel in the first place, it will be better than a series process.

Most "traditional" computer processes are automated, outdated and dependent series processes that have simply been moved from paper into a computer. The "new" processes are exactly the same as the old ones except that the bottlenecks are now hidden from sight "inside" a computer. It is no wonder that automation often makes things worse! Automation, however, can make things better. Computers can enable creative process improvement.

One must look for opportunities to creatively "parallel" around bottlenecks using computers. Freeways, for example, bypass bottlenecks by adding parallel lanes. Computers offer the same kind of opportunity to bypass bottlenecks by adding remote terminals (additional lanes) that can be used to parallel around bottlenecks. Computers can also perform bottleneck activities faster and, if needed, continuously. The place to begin managing bottlenecks is to find which "bulbs" have burned out and then "create" a parallel process around them, speed them up or keep them working full time.

In the series lights case, the bottleneck is hidden. How does the situation differ when the bottleneck is visible? In the next example, *The Hike*, the effects of a "visible bottleneck," coupled with a second problem, statistical fluctuations, are illustrated.

The Hike: Visible Bottlenecks and Statistical Fluctuations

"Bottleneck tasks" contribute significantly to the high cost and poor quality inherent in all business processes. They slow everything down. The example of "series lights" illustrates the bottleneck task's impact on an entire process and can provide insight for doctors who are beginning to approach cost and efficiency problems.

While a bottleneck is always the primary problem in a process, there is another cost and quality problem inherent in all series business processes. This is statistical fluctuation or variance. The best way to illustrate the magnitude of this problem is to again use an example based on everyday experience. In his book, *The Goal,* Eliyahu Goldratt illustrated both bottleneck and statistical fluctuations by using the example of a Boy Scout troop's 10-mile hike. The scoutmaster of this troop calculated that if each scout averaged two miles distance per hour, the 10-mile hike would take the entire troop five hours to complete. When it took his troop the five hours just to reach the half-way point, he was puzzled. What had gone wrong?

The hike wound along a narrow trail that required the troop to walk in single file. The scoutmaster observed that an interesting pattern developed as the hikers progressed forward; spaces began to appear between groups. The largest group accumulated behind an overweight hiker named Herbie.

Chart one

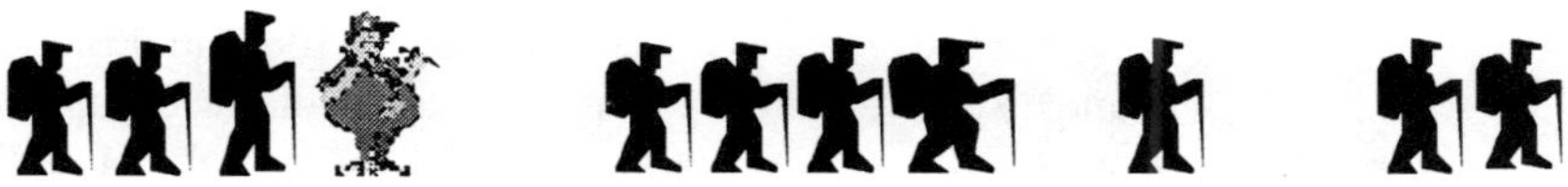

As the line continued to lengthen, the scoutmaster became concerned because he could no longer see the hikers at the front of the line. He relayed a message to the front demanding that the leaders stop and wait for the remaining hikers to catch up.

When all the hikers caught up with the front of the line, the scoutmaster asked that they attempt to stay together. The hike resumed, but at this point, the path widened, and the faster hikers were able to pass the slower ones, eventually leaving Herbie at the end of the line. There were no more groups accumulating, but the line began to lengthen even faster than before. The scoutmaster again relayed a message to the front of the line and asked that everyone stop in a group, maintaining the current order.

Chart two

He then asked all of the scouts to take hands and reverse the order of the line so that the slowest hiker would be at the front of the line and the fastest hiker at the rear. When they resumed hiking, Herbie was at the front of the line, and the troop stayed together in "tight formation" for the remainder of the hike.

Chart three

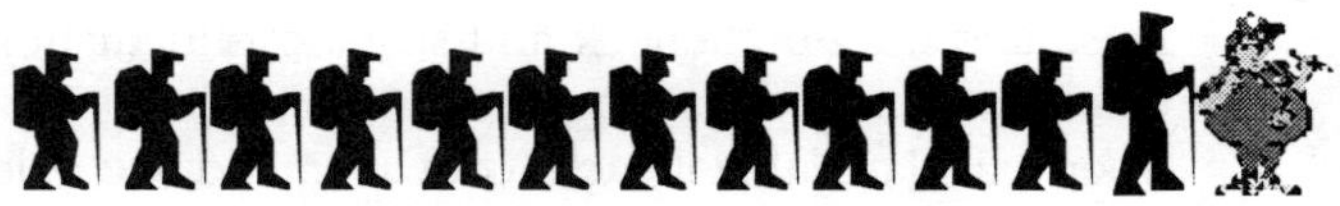

Many concepts can be learned from *The Hike*, and each one can help to form the foundation for analyzing and redesigning key processes within your office. The observations made by the scoutmaster during the hike represent statistical phenomena present in each process within our offices. Understanding these phenomena is one of the most important tools for lowering costs, increasing productivity and improving quality.

Hike Bottleneck

In the previous example, the scoutmaster's goal was that the entire troop arrive at the destination together. There was no advantage in having the fastest scout arrive first. In the initial phase of the hike (chart one), small accumulations of faster walkers grouped behind slower ones. The slower walkers should be thought of as the "bottleneck hikers." There were many of these bottlenecks when the hike was in a single-file series, and they were easy to spot because of the groups of hikers behind them.

In a manufacturing process, bottlenecks of this type are easy to spot because they appear as accumulations of "work in process" stacked in front of "bottleneck machines." If we are examining a paper process such as insurance billing, the bottlenecks are easy to spot because they show up as stacks of insurance forms or other papers on a desk. If we are evaluating a scheduling process, the bottlenecks show up during the busiest hours in the form of a line of people waiting at the front desk and phone lines being put on hold.

In the second phase of the hike (chart two), the line continued to lengthen, but with no separate groups of hikers. **There were no "visible" bottlenecks**. This is similar to a computer process where there are no "visible" stacks of paper to identify the bottlenecks. Even though the bottlenecks are not seen, they are there, just as before. Similar to the series lights example, there is only one bottleneck that controls the speed and efficiency of the entire troop. A bottleneck can be located anywhere within the process. In this phase of the example, the primary bottleneck is still Herbie, but he is now located at the end of the process and is, therefore, less noticeable.

The key to completing this task faster is to figure out how to make Herbie go faster. Similar to either manufacturing or business processes, the troop can speed Herbie up over the short term by eliminating waste. This could be accomplished by removing his heavy backpack and sharing its contents among the other hikers. Over the long term, however, Herbie can only be speeded up by getting him in shape (making him more efficient), and this takes time. Getting an inefficient office process into "shape" also takes time.

In the third phase of the hike (chart three), Herbie leads the troop and the line stays together. It is critical to recognize that **no matter where Herbie is located in the line, *he* controls the time it will take for the entire troop to reach its goal**. Any attempt to increase the speed of the troop is a waste of time and effort if it is focused on any hiker other than Herbie. Similarly, any attempt to increase the efficiency of a process in your office is a waste of time and money if it is not focused on the **primary** bottleneck. **The primary bottleneck controls the total time** (cycle time) **for completing the entire process, and eliminating any other bottleneck does not alter the cycle time**. This is why practitioners are often surprised when they invest money to "improve" their practice, and it doesn't show up on the bottom line.

Placing Herbie at the front of the line does create a better process in the sense that the line is easier to manage when set up in this order. In business, this could translate into less cost because there is less management supervision required. This does not improve the overall efficiency of the process, but it does lower the cost and complexity of management supervision, the principal focus of recent downsizing in corporate America. Also, if the bottleneck is at the front of the process, it is easier to focus on finding solutions for eliminating it.

The goal of Continuous Quality Improvement (CQI) is to make the "Herbies" faster. If Herbie joined a health club during the summer and lost weight while gaining strength, he would no longer be the primary bottleneck. The next slowest hiker would be the new bottleneck, and using Continuous Quality Improvement techniques, the scoutmaster would now attempt to "improve" this second scout. **CQI means always looking for the next bottleneck and working to "fix" it**.

Hike Analysis

When analyzing the hiking process, the scoutmaster realized that it consisted of a dependent series of activities. If each scout averaged two miles an hour, he sometimes walked faster than two miles an hour (say, two-and-a-half miles per hour) and sometimes slower (e.g., one-and-a-half miles per hour). This fluctuation around the average is referred to as variance, and in this case, the variance can be expressed as two miles plus or minus one-half mile per hour (2 ± 0.5 miles per hour). When the variances (the pluses and minuses) for an individual hiker are taken into account, he comes out with an average speed of two miles an hour. The scoutmaster incorrectly assumed from this that the individual variances would average out evenly for the entire troop over the entire hike.

The reason that statistical fluctuations do not average out for the entire troop is that the hike is a **dependent** series of activities. A scout's ability to walk faster than his average speed is constrained by the speed of the person walking immediately in front of him; however, there is no constraint on his, or any other hiker's, ability to walk slower than average. Therefore, it is impossible for the variances to average out in the same way that they would if an individual were making the hike by himself. **The negative variances accumulate throughout the entire process, and *an accumulation of slowness* results**. This accumulation has the side effect of causing the line of hikers to lengthen, making the process more difficult for the scoutmaster to supervise.

It is important to understand that this kind of accumulation of slowness is unknowingly designed into our business processes. Just as in the example of the hike, this accumulation is beyond the direct control of the employees working within the process. This is why most of our office processes take twice as long as their designers think they should, even when the processes are working "perfectly." Unfortunately, those who design processes blame poor performance on employees rather than on the processes that they (the designers) have developed. Simply having employees work harder cannot improve or change an inefficient process.

We have all experienced this "accumulation of slowness" on freeways. Often, the traffic in front of our car comes to a complete stop for no apparent reason. The actual cause might be an accumulation of negative fluctuations created by a car slowing (not necessarily stopping) far ahead. A negative variance accumulates throughout the system until, at some point, traffic comes to a stop. Understanding the cause of this problem has powerful applications to the solutions of many front and back office inefficiencies.

Assume that a business process, such as billing, consists of 10 linked steps (though it actually can have a lot more). The process begins with marking a superbill and ends with depositing a check. If one were to measure the average time it took to perform each of these 10 steps within the process, it would be discovered that the entire process actually takes at least twice as long as might be predicted from totaling the individual times for each of the 10 steps. If there are any "special" problems, such as an absent employee or a "computer glitch," the process will take even longer. While employees within the process can work to reduce or eliminate "special" problems, they have no control over the accumulation of negative variances ("common problems"). Common problems are often invisible, and it takes statistical methods to find and reduce them.

As is the case with bottleneck problems, the accumulation of negative variances adds cost and reduces the effectiveness of an entire process. As you might recall, the bottleneck problem can be solved by creating a parallel process to increase capacity at the bottleneck point. Negative variances can be reduced by eliminating unnecessary steps. Elimination of unnecessary steps reduces both the time needed to perform an activity and the additional variances created by that activity. This means that it is possible for fewer employees to do a better job! If fewer people can complete the billing process faster and better, profit is increased by reducing the total cost of salaries, and revenue is increased by increasing the collection ratio of the billing process.

Cost-reduction and quality improvement are the keys to future competitiveness and profit improvement. Speeding up bottleneck steps and reducing the number of tasks within a business process are powerful tools for quality improvement and cost-reduction, especially when applied to critical processes within the business office. The best method to achieve these goals is to improve and reengineer processes by creatively eliminating unnecessary tasks and increasing the capacity of bottleneck tasks.

The Freeway and Cycle Time

A busy freeway or highway combines the statistical problems of the hike and the series lights examples. It is important to understand the way a freeway functions because it has all the same problems that your office and clinical business processes do. The problems of a freeway, however, are more visible. If you understand the problems of freeways, you will be well on your way to understanding and solving the problems that are "hidden" in your business processes. These are the problems that create the high cost and inefficiencies that make it difficult for you to adapt to the changes brought about by managed care.

We have discussed the phenomenon that occurs on freeways when cars slow to a stop and then proceed forward with no visible sign of obstruction. This is a result of statistical fluctuations and the subsequent accumulation of slowness. As with the hike, for a car to average 55 miles an hour, it will sometimes go faster and sometimes slower than 55. If the car ahead is averaging the same speed, only the negatives accumulate. If the variance is small, say 55 ± 6 miles per hour, the car gets to where it's going, but it averages less than 55 miles an hour. If the variance is great (say a car slams on its brakes and slows to 30 miles an hour), each succeeding car reacts around this variance and, ultimately, cars farther back come to a stop. In this case, with a number of such variances, the total travel time for the individual cars on the freeway increases dramatically, and many of them are late arriving at their destinations.

The greater the number of cars on the freeway, the more the effect is magnified because each car has an individual variance that it contributes to the system. This is an important factor to consider when evaluating process steps. **Each activity adds both the time it takes to complete that activity and its variance**. Getting rid of unnecessary activities is an especially helpful step in becoming efficient because this eliminates the time required to complete those activities, their negative variances and the managerial supervision associated with them. Statistical fluctuations will always make a project take longer to complete (often much longer) than one would predict from simply adding the times required for all the individual tasks within the project. This is true, even when each task is accomplished "perfectly," because of the influence of accumulated negative variances. We need a strategy for dealing with such fluctuations and for preventing the complications arising from them.

A final example of this variance phenomenon is one that I recall seeing on television many years ago. The producers of a program filmed a group of construction workers who were attempting to set a record time for construction of a house. The house took less than a day to finish! How is this possible when it took a full 16 months to complete a second-story addition to my house? To achieve this record time, the construction workers had to eliminate unnecessary activities, reduce variances between each project step to a minimum and perform series project steps in parallel. They understood the lessons taught in the "series lights" and the "hike" examples.

When cars on freeways come to a stop as a result of statistical fluctuations, we refer to invisible obstructions; however, cars also slow down or come to a stop as a result of visible obstructions. These obstructions can be either fixed or random ones, and they usually appear, or are made worse, during peak traffic periods. Such obstructions are bottlenecks. The fixed ones are designed into the freeway system. One example of this is a point where a freeway narrows, causing a reduction in the number of lanes. Random bottlenecks are temporary obstructions, and they occur at such points as car accidents, objects that have fallen onto the freeway, construction sites and other randomly occurring "temporary" events.

The drawing below demonstrates a "fixed" structural bottleneck located in Irvine, Calif., This is a point where two major freeways merge. The time it takes a car to drive from Ventura to San Diego will be **controlled** by the Irvine bottleneck. If the volume of cars on the freeway falls below a certain maximum, cycle time (the total time that it takes a group of cars to make the trip from Ventura to San Diego) will be controlled only by the speed limit; however, when the volume of cars is increased beyond the capacity of the bottleneck, the cycle time for the trip is determined by that bottleneck. Adding lanes before or after the bottleneck cannot improve the efficiency of the freeway because it does not change total time (cycle time). Only adding lanes at the bottleneck can have the effect of speeding traffic at this point, and the addition of this parallel system will decrease the cycle time for all cars traveling between Ventura and San Diego.

FREEWAY

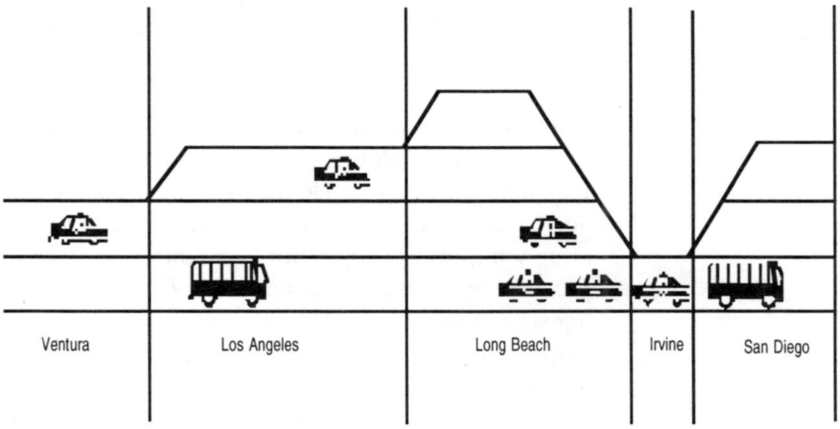

We observe this same type of bottleneck in our offices or clinics. The busier the day, the more bottlenecks surface. Some are fixed (which we unknowingly design into our processes), while others occur randomly as a result of such events as an absent employee or a computer breakdown. The location of fixed bottlenecks can be predicted in advance while random bottlenecks cannot. In order to make dramatic improvements in our office efficiency, we need a method for managing both types of bottlenecks.

The reason that eliminating bottlenecks is critical to solving cost and efficiency problems is that they control the cycle time for an entire process. Reducing cycle time is one of the most important keys to solving cost and productivity problems. With the example of the hike, the concept of the bottleneck (Herbie) was introduced and it was demonstrated how he controlled the speed of the entire troop. It is more difficult to make this same observation about seemingly unconnected tasks or events. Just as in the example of the hike, however, focusing on any activity other than the bottleneck will not improve the efficiency or cut the cost of an office process.

As in the hike, assume that "getting there together" is always an important feature. In an office, it is not important how long it takes for each individual task (such as filing each chart or entering data necessary to begin the billing process). The filing job is not completed until **all** the charts are filed, and the insurance cannot be billed until **all** data are entered.

Returning to the freeway example will help to clarify some of these ideas. While the freeway differs in that the goal is not that all cars arrive together, each car's cycle time is tied to the same bottleneck. For business purposes, cycle time has come to be defined as the total time required to complete a project. This "total time" to complete a project is what we ultimately want to reduce.

Another way to define cycle time is by stating a "number of units completed per hour." For example, if 10 insurance forms are completed per hour, the cycle time for completing insurance forms could be stated as 10 forms per hour. If changes have been made to "improve" the process, but the number of forms completed per hour has not increased, the primary bottleneck has not been identified.

The cycle time at the primary bottleneck (the slowest activity step in the process) determines the cycle time for the entire process. This means that the cycle time for the entire process cannot be decreased without first fixing the primary bottleneck. Spending time or money improving any other task makes no significant change in the process. For example, assume that cars are moving on a three-lane freeway at the rate of 210,000 cars an hour. At one point, the freeway narrows to two lanes, and one mile later, it again returns to three lanes. If the cycle time decreases to 30,000 cars an hour at the primary bottleneck (the point where the freeway narrows to two lanes), the cycle time for the entire freeway becomes 30,000 cars per hour. If this were a freeway from Los Angeles to San Diego, 30,000 cars per hour would arrive in San Diego no matter how many lanes were in place after or before the bottleneck and no matter what the speed limit was.

The total time it would take an individual car leaving Los Angeles to arrive in San Diego would be influenced by the bottleneck only when the freeway carried more than 30,000 cars an hour. There could never be more than 30,000 cars per hour arriving in San Diego unless the primary bottleneck was fixed.

It is clear that spending money to add more lanes in front of or after a bottleneck will not help, but this type of "improvement" is done all the time. Adding lanes helps cars to arrive at the bottleneck sooner, but it does not change cycle time and it does not decrease the total trip time for individual cars when freeway capacity exceeds 30,000 cars an hour. A few billion dollars could be wasted adding car pool lanes and synchronized on-ramps in front of the bottleneck if nothing is done about the bottleneck itself. All of this effort and money would not change the cycle time; however, investing only a few million dollars to add a third lane at the one-mile bottleneck stretch would change the freeway cycle time from 30,000 cars back to 210,000 cars an hour, a seven-fold increase!

Up until now there has been no direct connection made between automobile speed and cycle time. However, once a bottleneck is "fixed," increasing speed decreases cycle time. Increasing speed will continue to decrease cycle time up to the point that the capacity of the next bottleneck is reached. Again, using the freeway example: If a new bottleneck occurred at a point where traffic flow was reduced to 150,000 cars an hour, this would become the new cycle time, and a new bottleneck would need to be eliminated. Once a bottleneck is fixed, there is always another one to overcome. This is why Continuous Quality Improvement becomes important after reengineering has been completed.

An article entitled "Smart Highways, Foolish Choices?" appeared in the Nov. 28, 1994, issue of *Business Week*. This article presented a case for automating highway systems to eliminate the need for new roads by making it possible for cars to move faster and be spaced more closely. "Specially equipped cars would travel at high speeds, closely bunched, under the control of computers that are on board, along the roadside, and at a regional control center."

One researcher estimated that this would cost $75 billion for 5,000 miles of roadway, and the Department of Transportation announced that it was funding a $200-million, seven-year project. While this may sound far-fetched, a few far-sighted individuals are using cycle time principles to try to solve highway problems. If the projected cost of automating highways is less than the cost of new road construction, automation may come to fruition. Business process problems can be addressed in the same manner, and there are creative and less costly ways that technology can be applied to solve these "smaller" problems.

When you begin to make changes in your practice, it will be important to occasionally step back and rethink the points made in the series lights, the hike and the freeway examples. Experts that you might hire, including computer experts, often do not understand these principles. You will need to be able to evaluate technology (or any other device that is supposed to improve productivity or cut costs) from the standpoint of, "Does this eliminate the primary bottleneck and reduce cycle time?" We can add to this, "Does this eliminate unnecessary activities?" If the answer is "yes," we need to learn how to quantify the cost versus the benefit of making the change.

Cycle-time reduction is important to learn because it is not simply a matter of time measurement. **There is a direct correlation between cycle time, customer satisfaction, quality and increased profits**. Other industries have paved the way in using these principles, and this is precisely the strategy that medical practitioners need to compete profitably under managed care.

Regarding the issue of quality, Solectron Corporation reduced defects from 100 parts per million to 2 parts per million by reducing cycle time. Iomega cut its production cycle from 28 days to a day and a half by focusing on cycle time. Motorola reduced defects from 150 per 100 televisions to 4 defects per 100 televisions using cycle-time reduction and quality management techniques. These techniques will be covered later in this book.

Fred Wenninger, CEO of Iomega, stated that, "The cycle-time approach can be applied to paperwork procedures as well .... I'm not sure you need anything else." Reengineering paperwork procedures will be a significant area for cutting costs and improving quality in a medical office or clinic, and this will be covered in detail later. The principles that apply to paperwork apply equally well to improving the quality and lowering the cost of every treatment process and "people" process throughout a medical practice.

Most doctors would agree that patient satisfaction is important, but they may be unaware of its connection to cycle time. Companies in other industries that have undergone restructuring to lower cost and increase quality have learned that they must become "customer focused." When a company makes changes to reduce cost and improve efficiency, it is to its competitive advantage that it be able to accomplish these changes in areas that are most valued by its customers. "Customer focus" and "cycle-time reduction" are synonymous terms. Focusing on cycle-time reduction leads to customer satisfaction.

In addition to eliminating bottlenecks and reducing statistical fluctuations, eliminating wasted activities also plays a significant role in cycle-time reduction. In the example of the freeway, wasted activities can be represented by excess numbers of cars on the freeway at any given time. If car pools and incentives for drivers to use different times of day for travel result in fewer cars on the freeway, statistical fluctuations will have less impact and there will be fewer opportunities for bottleneck points to exceed capacity.

Uncovering Hidden Waste in Your Practice

Following bottlenecks and statistical fluctuations, waste is the next most important cause of poor quality and high cost. As mentioned before, eliminating wasted activities also eliminates the fluctuations associated with those activities. Waste can be defined as any activity that does not add value for the "customer," which in medicine's case includes patients, employers, referring physicians and managed care organizations.

Detecting waste is critical when evaluating a practice because reducing waste can improve productivity far beyond what cost savings alone can accomplish. Waste has been found to be inversely related to the level of service quality. Eliminating waste not only makes an office more efficient and saves cost; it also improves the quality of medical services provided.

Several obstacles stand in the way when attempting to identify waste in a service business. First, waste is not easily recognized because it is usually disguised as extra "process" steps that appear to be necessary. Second, and more insidious, many wasteful and obsolete business practices are still being advocated by "experts."

The search for waste in my office began when I innocently picked up a chart and asked, "Why do we file insurance forms in the chart?" The answer was, "In case we need to resubmit the insurance. Plus, we need a record of it." My next question was, "Don't we have a record of the insurance form in the computer which we could generate if we need to resubmit a claim?" The answer was, "Yes, but it is easier to do it this way." I then replied, "But this process requires that you separate the copies, locate the chart, transport the chart, punch holes in the insurance form, open the chart, insert the form and then refile the chart."

Simple math showed me that this was, at least, a nine-step process which also had the unpleasant side effect of making charts unnecessarily thick and shelves overcrowded. I then asked, "Do we file a copy of the superbill in the chart for the same reason?" The answer was, "Yes." I then inquired, "Isn't this information also stored in the computer?" Again, the answer was, "Yes." Because the superbill was not filed in the chart at the same time as the insurance form, I deduced that I had now identified 18 wasted steps. Add another five steps for the explanation of benefits and every other useless piece of paper that found its way into the chart. The clincher was that when I pointed this out, I was told that we didn't have a problem because we had hired an additional full-time employee to do filing! This simple exercise identified two problems: (1) we did not trust our computer so we ran a parallel paper system; and (2) it is difficult to distinguish productive work from nonproductive work.

To carry this example further, the chart that I had picked up belonged to a diabetic patient who had come to the office for routine preventative care visits every six weeks over an eight-year period. When I calculated how many wasted hours had been spent filing useless paper in this one chart over those eight years, it came to 11 hours and 56 minutes, probably more time than I had spent treating the patient. But this was only the "tip of the iceberg."

My next task was to follow the movement of the chart through the office during a single patient visit. First, it was "pulled" the evening prior to the visit and transported to the front desk. There it was opened, a blank treatment sheet inserted, and a date stamped on the treatment sheet. On the following day, when the patient arrived, it was moved to the end of the desk to signal that the patient was waiting for a treatment room. The chart was then transferred to the back office and later placed in a slot to signal that the patient was ready for the doctor. The doctor then transported it to the treatment room where notes were recorded in it before it was carried to the billing desk a considerable distance away. The chart would then be transferred to a "to-be-filed" pile and later refiled. This process included 13 steps, 12 of which were waste. Over eight years, this chart has gone through 2,496 wasted steps. As you might expect, this was not the end.

I have always manually marked this particular patient's diagnoses and services on superbills. These data are later entered into the computer by another person, duplicating at least three of the steps I have already completed. When the patient leaves the office, she waits to speak with the receptionist at the front desk to schedule her next appointment. To accomplish this one task, the receptionist must stop, put the phone on hold, inquire as to the nature of the next appointment, schedule the appointment and fill out an appointment card. She may even continue a conversation with this patient while a second patient is waiting on hold. This appointment could have been made more efficiently by a person in the back office who was already familiar with the patient's most current clinical needs. The eight-year wasted-step total for this one chart is now 2,912. This figure is relatively small; patients requiring more complicated services present even more opportunities for wasted steps.

Because so much waste of this type is present in most practices, solving "the waste problem" presents a practitioner with numerous opportunities for decreasing costs and raising quality. It also presents opportunities for turning wasted activity time into productive work time.

Total Quality Management: Lower Costs with No Sacrifice in Quality

Total Quality Management (TQM) has come to be associated with the return of U.S. manufacturing firms to a new competitive level. Despite the potential for similar gains in the services sector, the health care industry has been slow to incorporate TQM principles. These techniques can be successfully applied to a medical practice to lower cost without lowering quality.

Given the current highly competitive environment, some practitioners and institutions will not survive. I am convinced that TQM and reengineering methods will make the difference between success and failure in a medical practice, a clinic, an HMO, a hospital, or an educational institution. No matter what form the health care industry ultimately takes, higher quality and lower cost will become increasingly important.

One reason the health care industry has been slow to adopt TQM is that its diverse concepts are difficult to apply. Also, a quality service is harder to define than a quality product. Some TQM concepts include: teamwork, cross-training, continuous learning, continuous improvement, elimination of waste, elimination of bottlenecks, customer focus, employee autonomy, cycle-time reduction and group problem solving. Many of these concepts will work only when applied in a "commitment" environment rather than an old-fashioned "control" one. This is especially important in a medical practice, because doctors are occupied by treating patients and have little time to supervise or "control" employees working in the business office. These employees must be able to act independently, and this requires commitment.

The most important use of TQM is to identify actual problems in order to implement the proper solutions. A "proper" solution is one that raises quality and lowers costs. (Later, working toward the elimination of bottlenecks and waste will be discussed as being a cost-effective method for solving "actual" problems.)

Because the identification of the correct problem is so important to making successful decisions, it needs to be reemphasized. Identifying the "wrong" facts will often lead to the wrong solution just as the wrong surgery, even if performed well, will lead to a bad result. Business schools teach case studies of companies that have instituted TQM methods. A classic successful case is that of the Florida Power & Light Company (FP&L). An article in *Across the Board*, June 1992, (a management magazine) illustrates the problem of focusing on the wrong facts and uses FP&L as its example.

FP&L leaders felt they had been successfully implementing TQM principles and were preparing a visit to their mentor, Kansai Electric, in Japan. FP&L leaders were excited because they felt they had "solved" a serious problem. They had greatly reduced the time it took to repair boiler tube leaks, thus minimizing the time the utility would be shut down when a leak occurred. They were hoping to impress executives at Kansai Electric by showing them how quickly they could repair their leaks. When FP&L representatives asked the executives at Kansai how long it took them to repair leaks, Kansai executives did not understand the question. At first, the FP&L executives thought their question was lost in translation, so they continued to ask it in different ways. Eventually, the interpreter, translating a reply from the Kansai executives, asked, "Why do your tubes leak?" Kansai had found a method for preventing leaks; they didn't need to shorten the time needed to repair them!

Similarly, practitioners spend a lot of time and money fixing the wrong problems because they are focusing on the wrong facts. Individual offices have pieced together processes over the years to "fix" various problems as they occurred. Many elaborate processes have been put together by focusing on the wrong facts, processes that are rife with waste and bottlenecks. The computerizing of offices is an example of this. Many doctors have spent a great deal of time computerizing their offices and have neither increased quality nor lowered cost by doing so. The processes within these computers are often not improved ones but are merely the same old paper processes being performed on an electronic screen.

In my office, the search for "correct facts" began when I asked the question, "Why do we file these in the charts?" This question led to the discovery of an important bottleneck. Another of our office bottlenecks was that data from the superbill were not being entered into the computer until the following day. We asked the question, "How do we eliminate this delay in data entry?" Kansai executives might have asked, "Why do you need to enter this data twice?" After all, the doctor has already marked the diagnosis and charges; once should be enough. As we analyzed other processes, from scheduling to people movement, similar discoveries were made.

It is current practitioners, attempting to make a living in this highly competitive environment, who have the most to gain by applying TQM and reengineering methods. As soon as they begin, they will be well on the road to finding the answer to the question, "Why do your tubes leak?"

CHAPTER

4

Basic Analytical Tools

Electronic Spreadsheets for Data Analysis

The important information that FP&L gained from Kansai executives was that they needed to use correct facts and "ask the right questions." The electronic spreadsheet is an essential tool for assisting in collecting correct facts (data) and asking the right questions. While the typical businessman is never more than an arm's length from an electronic spreadsheet, few doctors use them.

One of the problems associated with a changing industry is the lack of data necessary for use in predicting how best to prepare for the future. This is true for the changing health care industry, but conveniently, data useful for addressing efficiency problems to be faced under managed care is already present in your office computer and can be directly downloaded onto an electronic spreadsheet. Even if you are not computerized, relevant data can be entered manually onto a spreadsheet in a short time.

There are many types of electronic spreadsheets on the market, and they are all adequate for our needs. Using a training manual, the basic functions of a spreadsheet can be learned in about eight hours. Advanced features require more time to learn, but they are not essential for most common problems.

An important feature of spreadsheets is that they free the user from tedious, repetitive calculations, thus providing greater insight into what the numbers are actually doing, what is driving them and how different assumptions about the future might affect them. Instant recalculation of all relevant numbers on a spreadsheet is achieved when any individual number on the spreadsheet is changed. These numbers also can be converted instantly into graphs that allow easy visualization of trends and the relative magnitudes of changes.

When "numbers crunching" is completed, the original spreadsheet can be preserved to be used again and again. At the same time, each change that you wish to save can be kept as an additional spreadsheet simply by giving it a different name. As you create multiple spreadsheets, they can be easily linked together to provide new information.

For doctors, the most useful basic feature of a spreadsheet is the opportunity it gives to ask "What if?" questions. The important information needed for this kind of question is data and assumptions pertaining to cost, volume and revenue. Once a spreadsheet is established, these data are entered and can be altered in various ways to see resultant effects on profit. For example, the risk of a contract can be evaluated by quickly determining which variables will affect profit the most and how sensitive profit will be to a range of assumptions (guesses) regarding variables such as price, utilization and cost. In the future, the same spreadsheet can be reused to evaluate the same type of contract without having to set it up again.

I might wonder how a proposed change in the Medicare fee schedule would affect my practice. Assume that Medicare will be raising evaluation fees by 5 percent, lowering surgical fees by 20 percent and restricting return visits to eight-week intervals. If I had previously established a spreadsheet, I could enter the new fees and immediately quantify the effect that these changes would have had on my practice last year. I would know whether my income would have gone up or down and by how much. If the spreadsheet calculates a decline of $13,480, I would have now quantified the direction and magnitude of the potential problem and would be in a much better position to begin solving it. For one thing, I already know how much I will have to reduce my costs ($13,480) if I wish to maintain my current salary under the new fee schedule.

I might now ask the computer, "What volume increase do I need to offset the decline in profit predicted by the Medicare fee changes?" I could play "What if?" by altering volume numbers up and down (both surgical and nonsurgical) and observing the resultant effects on revenue and profit. Again, I would immediately obtain necessary volume numbers, and I could evaluate whether the increase in volume was feasible. During such a process of entering data and watching resultant changes, you can gain a better understanding of the relationships in your practice among cost, volume and revenue, and discover which changes impact profit the most.

Using a computer, you can also sensitivity-test proposed solutions easily by examining how well each holds up as underlying assumptions are changed up or down to reflect "best case" or "worst case" scenarios. This testing is riskless and costless, and the results of such testing will give you the confidence to face change. It is important to find out how sensitive your predicted profit is to small changes in your underlying assumptions regarding fees, volume and costs. For example, **a 2 percent decrease in cost might have the same effect on profit as a 10 percent increase in patient volume.** Which change would be easiest for you to effect? Whatever the answer is for your practice (it will be different for each one), with this information you will be in a better position to know where to focus your efforts.

One function of a spreadsheet that I have found useful is its capability of tracking the price sensitivity of noncovered services and products. One might ask how varying a case fee might affect volume and profit. As a case fee is increased, demand should decrease and volume should decline, but would profit go up or down? The answer is that it could do either. The following is the formula for profit:

$$\text{Profit} = (\text{Price} \times \text{Volume}) - \text{Cost}$$

$$\text{Profit} = (P \times V) - C$$

We know that when we raise a price, demand will decrease and volume will decline. Depending on the percentage that volume declines, profit could either go up or down.

Assume that, during last year, you averaged 20 visits for "service A" each month, with a case fee of $300. If the supply cost for each visit was $80, last year's profit for "service A" was $52,800.

$$\text{Profit} = [\$300 \times (20 \times 12)] - [(20 \times 12) \times \$80]$$

$$\text{Profit} = \$72{,}000 - \$19{,}200$$

$$\text{Profit} = \$52{,}800$$

Assume that you raise the case fee to $350, and during the first three months following the fee increase, volume drops to 18 "service A" visits a month. Using the formula above, the predicted annual profit would be $58,320 instead of $52,800 (a $6,320 increase). In this case, you are seeing fewer service A visits, but your profit has increased. The goal should never be to achieve the maximum number of visits possible; it should be to achieve the **optimum** number (the number that produces the most profit).

Every fee change should be tracked carefully to follow its potential impact on volume and profit, and the spreadsheet can help you to do this easily for every service that you provide. Using a spreadsheet makes it possible to track monthly volumes and compare your numbers to historic values, thereby informing you of how much your volume and revenue are increasing or decreasing. At the same time, the spreadsheet can automatically enter totals into the formula above to predict a profit number. With this number, you can set a plan of action. If profit decreases when a fee is increased, the fee should be decreased or left where it is, but if profit increases when a fee is increased, your fee might still be too low.

If one were to attempt to do all of these calculations and trial scenarios manually, it would require too much time, there would be too many opportunities for mathematical and transposition errors and the dynamics of what the numbers are doing would be lost easily. Even for a simple problem, such as a single fee change, that new number would have to be multiplied by each procedure affected by the change, per month, and then these numbers would have to be totaled. This would have to be repeated manually for each single change in volume, price and cost. The focus would be on adding, subtracting, multiplying and checking for math errors rather than on learning strategic information. This type of "number crunching" does not stimulate creative thinking. Sensitivity testing to reduce risk would become too time consuming using this outdated method.

The questions that you might "ask" a spreadsheet are only limited by your ability to think creatively. I believe it was Ben Franklin who said, "A problem well stated is a problem half solved." This can be implemented with spreadsheets. Simply entering data and playing "What if?" immediately "states the problem well" and stimulates creative thought which, in turn, leads to better solutions—better because these solutions are focused on the correct problems. Relying on intuition or other nonquantitative techniques often can lead to identification of the wrong problems.

Before making any changes in your practice, test possibilities first by "playing with the numbers" on an electronic spreadsheet. This will quantify your problem, help you to understand the causes of the problem, lead you to possible solutions and allow you to test possible solutions by varying assumptions before investing any time or money in them. While making a decision will always involve some risk, a spreadsheet will help you to contain that risk.

Distinguishing the "Vital Few" from the "Trivial Many"

Time is a scarce resource, and we need to use that resource effectively. The most productive use of our time is to spend it focusing on issues in order of their priority. Given the amount of data that bombards each of us daily, it is difficult to differentiate important information from trivial information. Vilfredo Pareto (1848–1923) was a French-born economist who discovered that in most situations a small proportion of causes are responsible for a disproportionately large portion of a result. This is referred to as the *80–20 Rule*; 80 percent of a result is driven by 20 percent of its "causes." According to this rule, a doctor could assume that 20 percent of his or her office costs account for 80 percent of what is accomplished by the office, or that 20 percent of the office business processes account for 80 percent of the office costs. For purposes of optimizing our time and effort when engaging in problem solving, it is important to identify and focus on the vital 20 percent of a problem.

A Pareto graph is a useful tool. It is a visual format whereby key data (the 20 percent that drives the rest) is visually prioritized in the form of a bar graph arranged in order of the relative importance of data. The Pareto graph is a good starting point for problem solving because it clearly directs one's focus toward the issue that should be given the highest priority. We will never have time to solve every problem, but using the Pareto concept will allow us to address 80 percent of our problems by focusing on only 20 percent of their causes.

The most difficult part of solving a problem is knowing where to begin. Before proceeding, the following case study should help to illustrate this difficulty.

CASE ONE: WHERE DOES THE MONEY GO?

Dr. Jones had done everything right. He had a great reputation. He was board certified, and he was on staff at the best hospitals. His practice had grown steadily over 20 years, and he had added two partners to help him manage the increasing patient load. One partner was added in 1982 and the second in 1991. Despite significant revenue increases between 1990 and 1992, the partners' share of profit was shrinking.

At the end of 1992, Dr. Jones became alarmed because he realized that although the practice was too busy for two doctors to manage, there was not enough income to support three. He noted that the year before adding the third doctor, the two partners had billed out $1,000,000, of which they had collected $800,000 (an 80 percent collection ratio) with expenses of $400,000. They split the remaining $400,000 profit equally, and both felt well-compensated for their efforts. Dr. Jones also noted that the group of three doctors had billed out $1,428,571 two years later and had collected $1,000,000 (a 70 percent collection ratio). Expenses had grown to $639,875, leaving only $360,125 for three doctors to split (a 40 percent drop in income for the two original partners). Dr. Jones understood that fees had decreased, but he had thought that patient volume and revenues had increased more than enough to offset the difference.

The doctor did not know where to start, but he knew that he had better act fast. He immediately eliminated two full-time positions. This instantly improved cash flow. There was more income for the doctors, but the patients' waiting time increased significantly, complaints began to rise and Dr. Jones felt rushed with his patients. The improvement in cash flow was short-lived. Just three months later, income again began to drop. Billing remained constant, but cash was coming in more slowly. Upon investigating, Dr. Jones found stacks of unfinished paperwork, and his staff told him that they had been unable to keep up after the two business office positions were eliminated.

The doctor asked two employees to work overtime for a short time while he investigated what he could do to increase profit without lowering quality. Office morale was dropping, and the temporary overtime payments dropped the partners' salaries even further. Dr. Jones and his partners first focused attention on the cost of medical supplies. They assigned one nurse to check the price of every supply and negotiate better prices. Over a one-month period, this nurse was able to achieve a 10 percent reduction in the total cost of medical supplies. In the meantime, Dr. Jones and his partners agreed that they would save money by not going out of town for medical education. They also changed accountants. This reduced their accounting bills by 20 percent.

Dr. Jones spent several days closely examining telephone bills and noted that many personal calls were made by employees, some of which were long distance. He calculated that he could reduce the phone bill by 10 percent if he instituted a rule that no personal calls could be made from the office. He also decided that he would no longer make charitable contributions. Office morale began to sink.

Patient complaints continued to increase, and several referring physicians expressed concern. The doctor learned that the nurse who ordered supplies was spending so much time comparing prices that she was unable to devote much time to patient care. Worse yet, revenues were beginning to decline because patients were unable to obtain appointments quickly, and they waited too long for care after they arrived at the office. The staff felt overworked, and the front office staff (who were working overtime) gave notice that they could only continue on this schedule for a few more weeks. They requested that the terminated positions be reinstated.

Dr. Jones went back to his office to contemplate the situation while he opened his mail. The first piece of mail he opened was his rent bill, and it was stamped "overdue." He immediately checked the accounts payable and found a month's worth of bills waiting to be paid. No one had had the time to do this. Dr. Jones opened the next letter. It was from a patient informing him that neither she nor her family would be returning for care. The third letter was from a referring physician who had not received a medical report on the status of a patient he had referred more than two weeks before.

Dr. Jones decided to ignore the remaining stack of mail; he sat and contemplated. Medical school had not prepared him for this. He felt that he had tried everything he could to cut costs. **Rather than increasing profit, he had only succeeded in lowering quality. He knew that he needed to make some decisions fast, but what options were open to him?**

This doctor is facing a serious problem. His profit is declining, and when he attempted to improve it, his patients suffered by receiving poorer service. Ultimately, this poor service will lead to even further declines in profit. Currently, the doctor is attempting to cut costs by spending less money. While it is important that money not be wasted, cost and volume are related and should be considered together.

The place to begin is to look at practice expenditures. Dr. Jones's income statement, which he received from his accountant, is printed on the following page:

Income Statement 12 Mos.	Ended Dec 31, 1992	
Total Fees Collected	**$1,000,000**	
Operating Expenses		
Advertising	$15,046	
Automobile	$17,156	
Bank Charges	$3,733	
Beeper	$2,118	
Computer Supplies	$3,608	
Contributions	$4,410	
Dues/Subscriptions	$11,366	
Equipment Rental	$3,400	
Insurance	$42,000	
Janitorial Service	$3,660	
Legal/Accounting	$10,860	
Licenses	$2,546	
Medical Supplies	$30,987	
Office Supplies	$15,349	
Outside Lab and Products	$52,361	
Outside Services	$3,026	
Parking	$4,781	
Patient Refunds	$3,630	
Pharmacy/Drugs	$1,820	
Photography-Medical	$588	
Pension Plan Expense	$3,400	
Postage	$5,120	
Professional Development	$4,200	
Penalties	$618	
Promotion	$3,400	
Rent	$117,043	
Repairs	$2,648	
Salaries	$249,616	
Taxes	$2,314	
Telephone	$15,028	
X-ray	$3,077	
Total Operating Expenses	**$639,875**	**63.99%**
Net Income	**$360,125**	**36.01%**

One problem with this "typical" income statement is that it contains too many categories (31 in this example), and it is easy to lose focus by "getting lost in the numbers." The following chart lists only the 12 largest categories from this income statement.

EXPENSE	DOLLARS
ACCOUNTING	$10,860
ADVERTISING	$15,046
DUES/SUBSCRIPTIONS	$11,366
INSURANCE	$42,000
MEDICAL SUPPLIES	$30,987
OFFICE SUPPLIES	$15,349
OUTSIDE LAB	$52,361
PARKING	$4,781
POSTAGE	$5,120
RENT	$117,043
SALARIES	$249,616
TELEPHONE	$15,028

Reducing the number of categories helps to provide focus, but there is still a problem with this income statement: the expense categories have been arranged alphabetically. Wouldn't it make more sense to have the categories arranged in the order of importance (dollar amount) utilizing a Pareto graph? The Pareto graph is a useful visual tool for providing focus in the order of importance.

There is not enough time available for us to solve every problem that confronts us each day. We must prioritize them so that we are focusing on the "biggest ones" first. This requires a method of separating the "vital few" from the "trivial many." The Pareto graph is useful for displaying the relative importance of problems and measuring the impact of changes.

A Pareto graph for the largest 12 expenses in this example appears below, and from this, one can easily "see" where the money of this office goes. The order of importance of expenditures becomes readily visible.

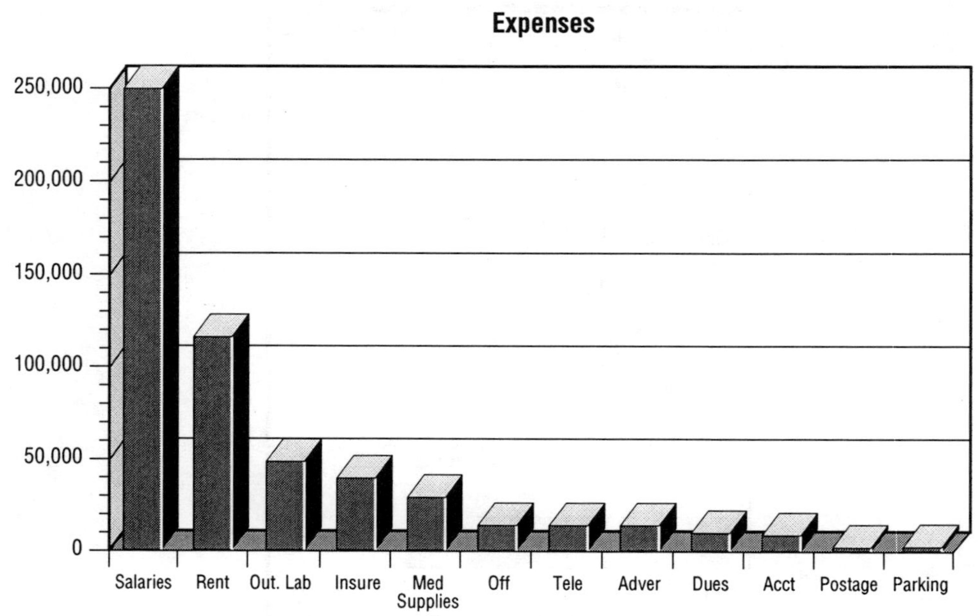

It is interesting to note that the top six expense categories represent only 20 percent of the total expense categories, but they account for 79.38 percent of total expenses. Earlier, we stated that it is efficient to reduce that problem to the 20 percent of issues that account for 80 percent of a problem. In this example, the Pareto chart accomplishes this task by demonstrating that 80 percent of this office's cost-associated problems can be attributed to 20 percent of the office's expense categories. This graph is more "strategic" than the accountant's statement.

Using the graph on the next page, it can be seen that given a limited amount of time, the doctor will get a "bigger bang for his buck" by focusing on reducing the cost of "Outside Lab and Products" before tackling the "Medical Supply" category. One could also conclude that time spent focusing on expenses such as the telephone bill or the cost of postage would detract from initiating the more difficult (but potentially more rewarding) task of reducing costs in the top six categories.

EXPENSES	DOLLARS
SALARIES	$249,616
RENT	$117,043
OUTSIDE LAB	$52,361
INSURANCE	$42,561
MEDICAL SUPPLIES	$30,987
OFFICE SUPPLIES	$15,349
TOTAL	$507,917

One significant "expense item" is still not reflected in the above chart. Our case stated that doctor Jones's collection ratio had dropped from 80 to 70 percent, resulting in $142,857 in lost income. This $142,857 might represent an inefficiency in the billing process, and this inefficiency will become more costly if patient volume grows.

If this reduction in the collection ratio were reflected as an "expense," a new, adjusted Pareto graph could be constructed to provide Dr. Jones with the best picture of where his money is going. The dollar-amount lost due to the decrease in the collection rate could be expressed as an "expense" on the Pareto graph. The doctor is now much closer to developing a focus and strategic plan for his future reengineering efforts. This adjusted Pareto graph appears below.

Adjusted Expenses: Pareto

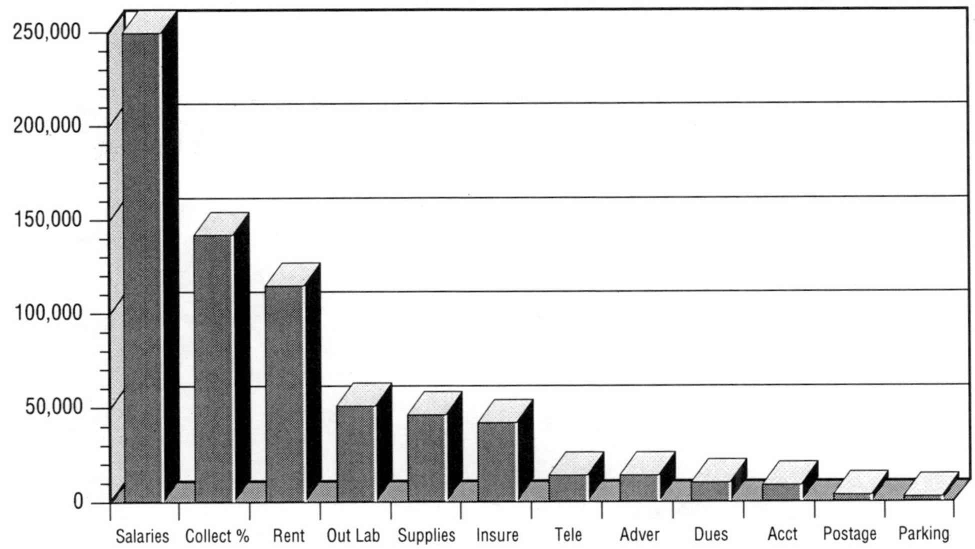

Dr. Jones has finally identified the relative importance of his key expense categories. This will help him formulate his strategic change plan. The three largest categories (Salaries, Collection Ratio and Rent) are also the most difficult ones to change because they all involve operational changes (probably reengineering) which will require training and involvement of the entire staff. This will also create a significant disruption in "normal" office operations. The next three categories (Outside Lab, Insurance and Supplies) are easier to change because the doctor can reduce cost by working alone with a calculator, paper, pencil, phone and fax machine. Cutting costs from the remaining expense categories should be delayed until the top six (the top 20 percent) are addressed.

Reengineering has a large payback relative to anything else the doctor can do. While it will require more time, more knowledge and more headaches, the final result can dramatically reduce cost, increase efficiency and position the doctor to compete profitably under managed care.

It is important to note that no costs are fixed over the long term. The doctor in this example is paying rent and salaries based on earlier decisions that were made using different assumptions regarding the marketplace and fee structure. At this time, he doesn't know whether more or less space, or more or fewer employees will be needed. The doctor doesn't know whether to consider sharing space, merging practices with another practitioner, or outsourcing business activities (such as billing to a billing service). He now knows where to focus his effort for the greatest return and won't waste time analyzing every supply cost and telephone charge.

Trend Analysis

It can easily be seen on the graph below (representing Dr. Jones's office) that each expense category in his office is moving upwards.

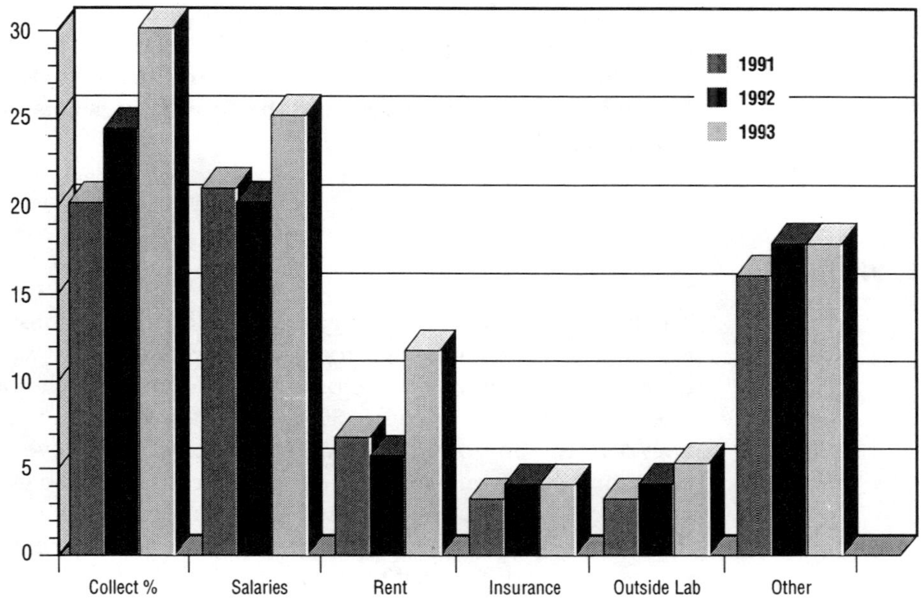

The collection ratio shows a significant problem between 1991 and 1993, which accounts for a substantial loss of income. **The graph does not explain causes, but it draws attention to important trends over time**. It is significant to know multiple-year trends for all important expense and revenue categories in an office. A computer can make this type of comparison fast, but it is necessary that the computer be used for this purpose over several years in order to build up an appropriate comparative database. Even if a practice is not computerized, transferring the accounts payable process to a "stand-alone" check writing system will automatically provide this data simply by using the computer to pay bills.

Before initiating any changes, Dr. Jones still needs more analytical tools. Cost-cutting sounds easy, but it is much like dieting. Just as "crash-diets" seldom result in permanent weight loss, "crisis cost-cutting" seldom results in permanent control over the causes of cost problems. To obtain the best results from either a diet or office cost-cutting, long-term strategies requiring increased knowledge and a **permanent** change in behavior must be implemented.

Dieting is not simply a matter of eating less. An effective dieter needs to be educated regarding the correct foods to be eaten and the proper amount and type of exercise to be undertaken. Similarly, cost-cutting is more than a simple matter of spending less. The quality of service can be hurt by cutting the wrong office costs just as malnourishment can be created by cutting the wrong foods from a diet. Information is required before taking action, as is knowledge of how to become both more efficient and more productive. **Streamlining work flow is the key to increasing efficiency, and the flowchart is a useful tool for analyzing work flow.**

Flowcharts

The flowchart concept was originally developed for improving the efficiency of manufacturing processes. It works equally well for analyzing the variety of office processes that make up the business operations of a medical office. A flowchart provides each individual who performs an isolated task within a process a bird's eye view of that entire process. It enables each person to see both the "bigger picture" and exactly how his or her individual task affects the final outcome. A flowchart helps a team to come up with ideas which might improve a process, and it assists that team in generating ideas for redesigning (reengineering) and "testing" new versions of that process **before** time **and money are committed to an improvement project.**

Various symbols are used in flowcharts, each depicting a certain type of activity. The activity is written within the symbol for purposes of analysis, but the total chart is what gives this bird's eye view. It is not important that traditional symbols be used, but a few of the more common symbols used in drawing flowcharts appear below.

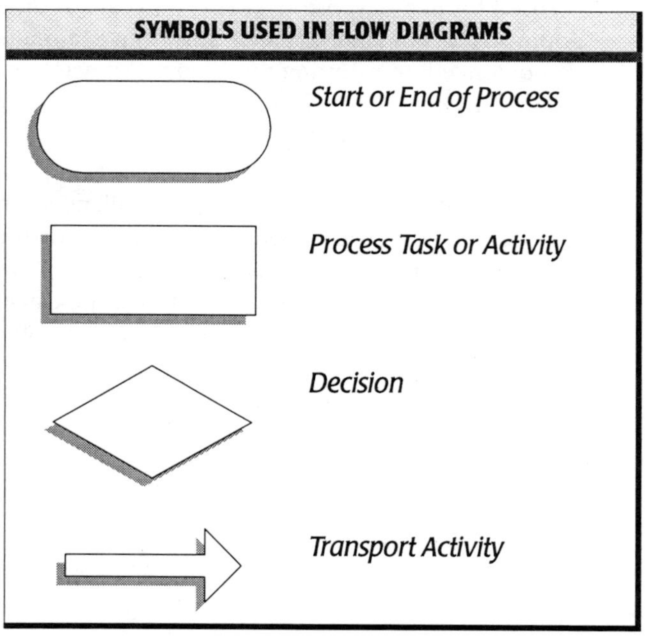

SYMBOLS USED IN FLOW DIAGRAMS (Continued)

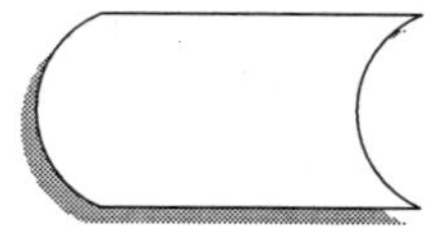

Wait

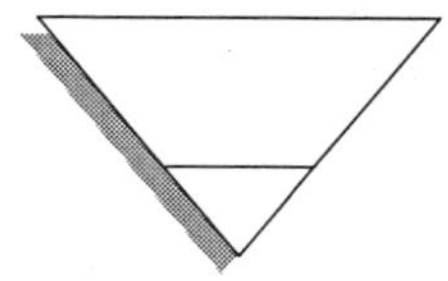

Storage

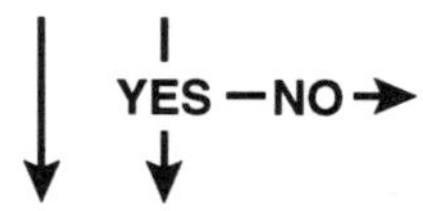

Next Activity

Developing a flowchart requires breaking a process down into its component tasks and then diagramming the work flow. To demonstrate how this is done, let us consider the relatively simple process of answering an office telephone. The phone rings, a person answers it, a patient asks a question, and someone answers the question. The receptionist draws a simple flowchart to depict this sequence of events:

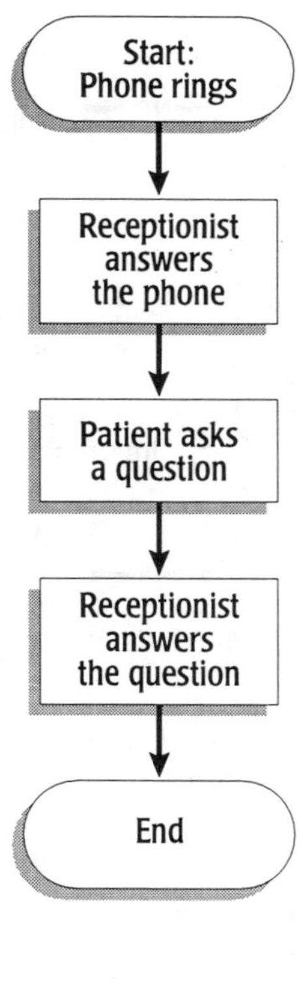

This flowchart represents the process steps and work flow as perceived by the receptionist. It can serve as a starting point for initiating dialogue and analysis directed toward understanding the process. A process cannot be changed for the better unless everyone performing that process first understands how it works.

When the doctor reviews this flowchart, he mentions that a process step is missing. He knows that patients often ask questions the receptionist is not able to answer. He asks, "What happens if you are not able to answer the patient's question?" The receptionist thinks about this and draws a revised flowchart that appears below.

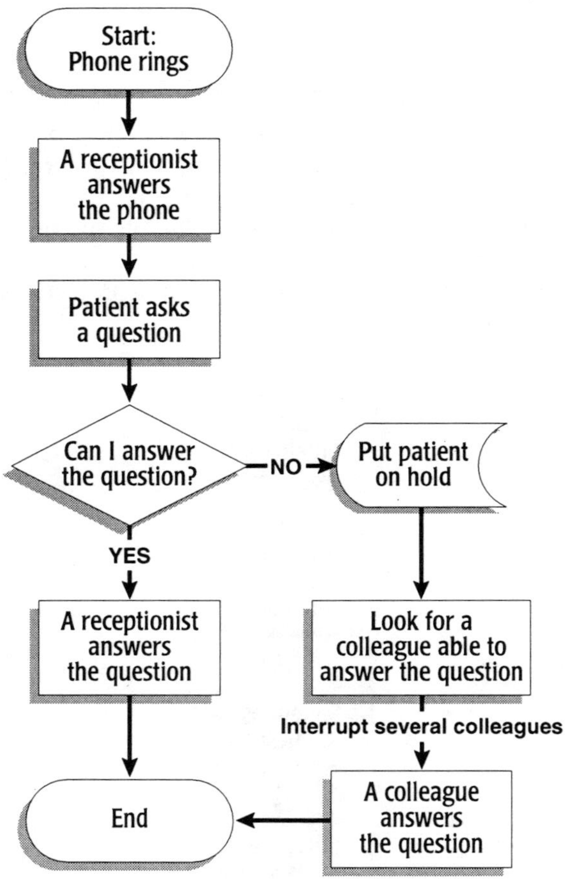

The revised flowchart is more complex than the first. The first change encountered in the revised chart is the "decision diamond" asking, "Can I answer the question?" If the answer is "yes," the work flow remains the same as before; however, if the answer is "no," additional process steps are added, making things more complex and thereby reducing efficiency. This will not only raise costs, but will also lower quality by making patients wait longer. **The answer "no" becomes the primary process bottleneck because additional wasted process steps and their associated variances are created as a byproduct**. Bottlenecks and wasted activities add cost with no corresponding benefit.

Quality becomes poorer as a result of this added step because the patient must now wait. Efficiency is poorer because the receptionist must leave the front desk, becoming unavailable for the next call, and other employees are interrupted and removed from productive tasks to perform the receptionist's work. Costs go up as a result of this extra work and inefficiency. If subsequent calls come in, each additional patient is put on hold, and this flowchart becomes even more complex.

It becomes obvious to the team analyzing the work flow that this process could be improved by eliminating the bottleneck and the wasted activities. The team decides that the "loop" appearing on the right side of the flowchart could be eliminated if the receptionist were given enough training to become autonomous and self-sufficient when answering the phone. Eliminating this loop improves the process in the following ways: 1) wasted activities associated with the search for another employee are eliminated; 2) interruptions of other employees who are performing productive work are eliminated; and 3) the number of patients who are placed on hold is reduced, with those patients who are put on hold being left there for a shorter period of time.

This process can be improved significantly by making a relatively simple change: the receptionist must be trained more thoroughly, and this is best done if she (or he) is cross-trained. The team was able to focus on the "correct" problem by understanding the process because of the flowchart. Whatever solution is devised by a team using a flowchart, it is more likely to be successfully implemented because everyone in the team better understands why the change needs to be made and is thus more likely to support the change. This "phone answering process" could be improved further, but at this point, we are limiting discussion to the use of a flowchart and not to solutions. **In this example, a noncritical process was improved but not radically changed (reengineered)**. Later chapters will discuss key processes (those that constitute 80 percent of an office's cost) and the decisions necessary for improving or changing (redesigning) those processes.

Customer Focus and Cycle Time

One key outcome in the example above was that the process of answering the phone became faster. This could be restated in the following way: **the cycle time for the process of answering the phone became shorter**. An important "byproduct" of this shorter cycle time is that the process of answering the phone becomes better for the customer too. The most important connection between cost and quality is that **when cost is reduced by shortening cycle time, the customer is always better off**. This can be stated in the following way: **reducing cost by shortening cycle time is a "customer-focused" cost-reduction**.

Customer focus is important to understand because there are many choices and tradeoffs to be made when reducing costs. The goal of cost-cutting should not be simply to improve profit; it should also be to improve quality. If the improvement in quality is in an area that is important to and valued by the customer, that cost-cutting will also increase the doctor's competitive advantage and create future opportunities for revenue generation through increased patient volume.

Customer focus becomes lost in most large companies because those companies are organized into functional departments. It is rare that one department or one person manages a complete process. Instead, most processes cross horizontally through several departments. There is someone in charge of each department, but no one is in charge of a complete process. When the people working within that process gather to improve or change it, they rarely focus on the entire process. Rather, they focus on the individual process tasks of their own departments and not on the process as a whole.

Focusing on individual process activities will never optimize the process as a whole; this, instead, results in "local optimization." Many of the process steps may be improved for the individuals performing those activities, but total process efficiency is not improved, and costs are likely to go up. This is comparable to adding freeway lanes in non-bottleneck areas. When functioning this way, bottlenecks are easily overlooked. The time delays between the completion of each individual activity and the start of the next cannot be "seen" by those who are performing those activities. Another problem is that money and time are often spent trying to improve activities that should be eliminated altogether.

A similar pattern is repeated in smaller medical offices and clinics, but it is less obvious. Usually, more than one individual is involved in a process; however, **individuals are rewarded for the outcome of their individual process tasks rather than on the outcome of the entire process**. They may improve (speed up) individual tasks, but this may only speed work to the bottleneck point. The process cycle time, and hence the cost and quality of the entire process, remains unchanged.

To further examine customer focus, let us look at the process of dictating letters (a simple and noncritical process). Assume that Dr. Smith dictates referral letters at the end of each day. In this example, she has three letters to dictate, and each one takes approximately five minutes to complete. In this case, the customers are the referring doctors.

The process steps consist of dictating the letters, removing the tape cassette, dictation service pick-up, typing the letters, returning the letters to the doctor, reading and editing the letters, copying and filing copies of the letters, stuffing the envelopes and mail pick-up. The chart below compares the processing times of the individual steps side by side with the cycle time for the entire process. In this example, the total processing time is 1 hour and 20 seconds while the total cycle time is 65 hours and 45 minutes.

		Processing Time	Cycle Time
5:00 p.m.	Dictate letters	15 min.	15 min.
5:15 p.m.	Remove cassette	10 sec.	10 sec.
12: 00 p.m.	Service pick-up	1 min.	18 hrs 45 min.
3:00 p.m.	Letter typed	30 min.	3 hrs 30 min.
12:00 p.m.	Letters delivered	5 min.	20 hrs 30 min.
4:45 p.m.	Doctor reads/edits	3 min.	4 hrs 45 min.
9:00 p.m.	Copy, stuff, mail	6 min.	15 hrs 51 min.
11:00 p.m.	Mail picked up	10 sec.	2 hrs 9 min.
Total		**1 hr 20 sec.**	**65 hrs 45 min.**

What is important is that the cycle time is 10 times greater than the processing time, and the time relevant to the customer is this total cycle time. The long cycle time is due to the considerable delay time between individual process steps. Two important observations can be made at this point. The first is that speeding up an individual task, such as typing or stuffing envelopes faster, will have little effect on the total cycle time. If the total processing time was cut by 50 percent, this would cut cycle time by only 30 minutes and 10 seconds. Cutting cycle time from 65 hours and 45 minutes to 65 hours and 15 minutes is of little value. **This is often the reason why so many offices are disappointed with their computers. They are using computers to cut processing time, not cycle time.** This, coupled with the increased complexity of the computer, often increases costs with no corresponding benefit.

It is helpful to draw the flowchart associated with this dictation process. It can be seen from the flowchart that even a relatively simple process can be more complex than it first appears.

LETTER DICTATION - FLOWCHART

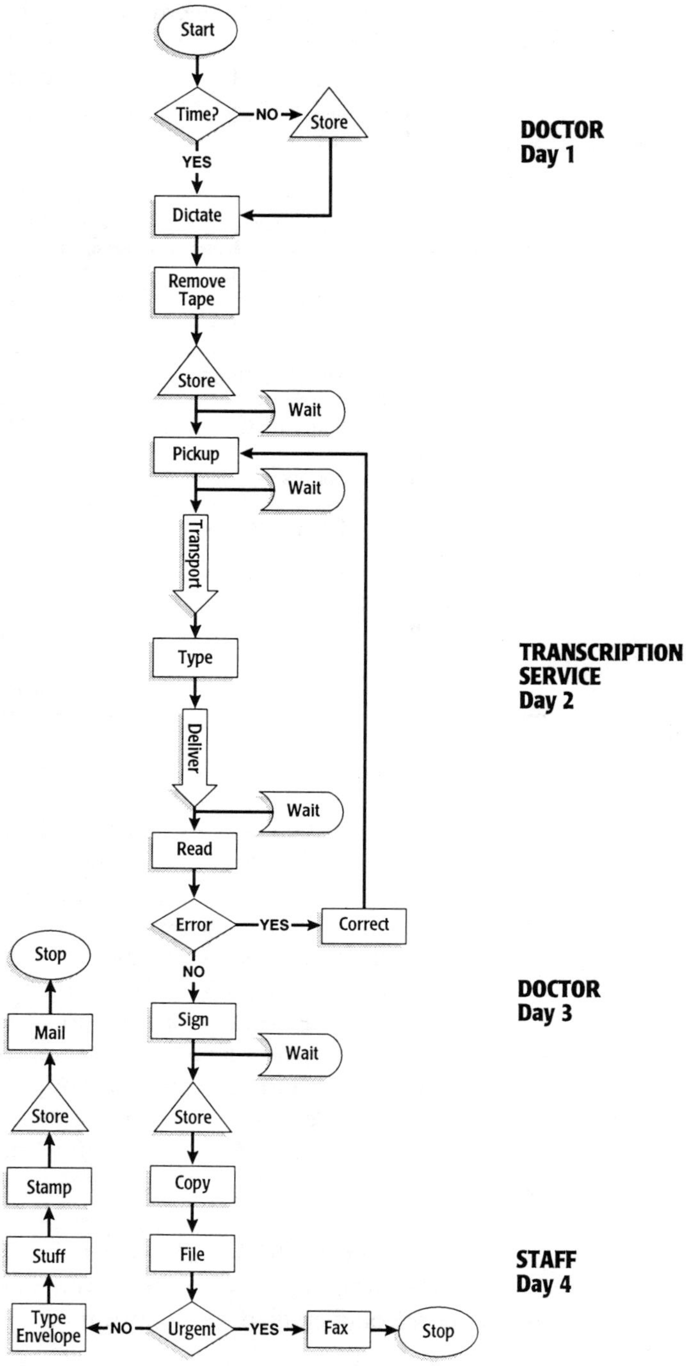

Each task within this process is being performed at a different time, on different days and often by different employees. Any individual employee who attempts to improve the process without involving other participants in the process will be unable to find the bottlenecks and the wasted activities, and without this as the goal, the process cannot be made more efficient.

We have not yet made allowances for statistical fluctuations (variances) in this example. Does the doctor dictate every night? What if she has a meeting and delays dictating until the following night? This adds 24 hours to the cycle time. What if she edits and returns the letter to be retyped? This adds another 24 hours to the cycle time. What if the office is busy or short-handed in the morning, and no one is available to stuff and stamp the letters at 9 a.m.? The 11 a.m. mail pick-up would be missed and another 24 hours would be added to the cycle time. Remember, none of these is an example of process breakdown; these are normal variations (statistical fluctuations) present in a process working precisely as it was designed to work.

Assume that this doctor receives a call from a referring physician who is irate because he has not received a report on a patient he referred 10 days ago. The doctor immediately explains to the referring physician that this is not possible because she knows that she dictated the letter 10 days earlier. Following this incident, she tries to find out who "slipped up." After all, it could not be her fault because she knows that it is her routine to dictate a referral letter on the same day that she examines a patient.

If this doctor had the relevant business skills, she would be able to determine that no one had "slipped up" and that the dictation process had worked precisely as designed. **Normal statistical variations, combined with a weekend, could easily add another six days to the process without the doctor "seeing" them**.

If this were a critical process, one that impacted cash flow or patient care, the doctor would need to "fix" it immediately. The skills needed to "fix" this noncritical dictation process are the same ones needed to fix critical processes that can result in dramatic efficiency improvements and cost-reductions. As always, with a focus on cycle-time reduction, the changes initiated will automatically be customer focused.

CHAPTER

5

Human Resource Development

Introduction

Before embarking on the chapters ahead, we will be taking a short break from the quantitative issues associated with change to discuss human issues. We are all familiar with the tendency people have to resist change or even subvert it. We are often afraid of the unknown and prefer to retain the status quo.

Changes that involve Business Process Improvement (BPI), quality management and reengineering will, at first, be disruptive; however, after taking the initial steps, positive changes will occur in the employees' work environment that will make their work both more interesting and more important. Organizing the office around processes rather than tasks takes much of the day-to-day decision making away from the doctor and gives it to the people located at the various points of service. Decision-making autonomy requires that each employee receive more education and training. This leads to employees who enjoy their work more. In this kind of environment, there is less employee turnover.

One of the main results of successful process improvement and reengineering is that an office or clinic will be more efficient and run better with fewer people. Many nonproductive activities will be eliminated. This does not necessarily mean that people will be laid off. There may be opportunities to turn previously unproductive work to more productive tasks directed at supporting a larger patient flow.

Two key ingredients required in an effective human resource policy are employee cross-training and employee empowerment. These are easy concepts to understand, but implementing them may not be as easy if "old-style management control" techniques are retained. The next few pages will help you understand what is meant by these terms, and later we will focus on how to convert these concepts into higher productivity and profit. If you make no changes in your office other than cross-training and empowering your staff, it will run more efficiently.

Employee Cross-training

There are two essential goals for both process control and management of people. The first of these is to create clarity and order, and the second is to facilitate learning. Later we will discuss how to create clarity and order by focusing on streamlining and simplifying processes. At this point, we will focus on the facilitation of learning. Ongoing learning is an essential feature in achieving continuous quality improvement. To achieve optimum productivity, it is important to discard some outdated ideas regarding job descriptions, motivation and training.

In a 1959 book, *The Motivation to Work*, Frederick Herzberg presented a strong argument that dissatisfaction is not the opposite of satisfaction. He showed that simply removing dissatisfying characteristics from a job did not necessarily make that job more satisfying or the employee more motivated. If such things as salary, office policy and working conditions are adequate, an employee will probably not be dissatisfied. He or she may not, however, be satisfied. In a study of more than 56,000 employees, "interesting work" was rated as the most important component of a job. Job descriptions tend to become more specialized and less interesting as a medical practice grows. This specialization not only tends to produce employees who are less motivated, it also creates much of the inefficiency, waste and higher costs that occur as a practice reaches maturity.

Eric Flamholtz, professor of human resource development at the UCLA Graduate School of Management, discusses three stages of organizational growth that apply well to the stages of development in a medical practice. These stages are: 1) starting a new venture; 2) rapid expansion of that venture; and 3) professionalization. He refers to the first two stages as the entrepreneurial phases of the business and the third as the professional management phase.

The reason this distinction is important is that entrepreneurial skills are quite different from those required of a manager in an organization that is in its "professional" stage of development. Unfortunately, a medical practitioner must have both sets of skills to be successful at all stages of a practice's development. The most common result of failing to make an effective transition into stage three is that profit will remain flat even as the practice continues to grow in both volume and revenue. **Growth of this type contributes only to work load, not profit**. Under managed care, practices enter stage three much sooner.

At stage three, an entrepreneur would continue to focus on marketing to increase revenue; however, what is needed now are professional management skills, those that increase efficiency. At this point, a professional manager recognizes the need for cross-training and teamwork, skills needed to curtail the increasing need for more employees.

When a doctor hires his or her first assistant, that assistant must learn every duty in the office from patient care to billing. Specialization begins when the office becomes busier, and a second assistant is hired. At this stage, one assistant typically works in the "front" office, and the other works in the "back." As each additional assistant is hired, his or her tasks become even more specialized. One becomes a receptionist, others become billing secretaries or chairside assistants. Each job becomes less varied and less interesting. Turnover and absenteeism increase, and employees are less motivated. Despite the fact that it would be better if all employees were trained to perform every duty in the practice, each new assistant now learns only a small part of the whole. This not only produces employees who are less motivated, it also leads to lower quality and higher costs. Why not reverse this process through cross-training? Consider the following example:

Various areas of the office are randomly busy. Eighty percent of a day's revenues might be generated during one two-hour period, just as 80 percent of a day's phone calls might occur during a different two-hour period. During these peak times, the options are: lose business, hire more people, or cross-train so that existing employees can be redistributed to where they are most needed during these peak periods. In addition, if an employee is absent, others can rotate to that position as needed to maintain productivity. The greatest gain from this kind of training is the continuous improvement that results because all employees now understand the "total" office. Each employee becomes more interested in identifying how to better serve the person next in line, the one who receives his or her completed work. Everyone has more knowledge to help identify bottlenecks occurring between different functional areas, and all employees are able to work better together in finding solutions to problems. Potential solutions are implemented more quickly because consensus already has been obtained from the individuals responsible for implementation. Ultimately, employees can be given greater autonomy to make decisions, something that previously required much of the doctor's time.

Facilitation of learning is an important goal of management that doctors already understand. There is nothing difficult in understanding management techniques such as cross-training and teamwork. In fact, most doctors start with these ideas, and as the office becomes busier, they tend to move away from them, just as their potential for "helping the practice" increases. Implementation of these techniques is not easy; however, the potential gains of higher quality, lower costs and a "happier" work environment are well worth the effort.

Employee Empowerment: A Few Good People

During a time of declining reimbursement rates, practitioners must take a closer look at cutting expenses. In Chapter 2, it was demonstrated how, as a profit margin narrows, cutting expenses can have a more profound effect on profit than increasing patient volume. The biggest expense item in a medical practice (often as high as 25 percent of revenue) is the line item "employee salaries." Because this is the area of greatest potential savings, it makes sense that it would be the first one a doctor examines when preparing to cut costs.

When I first entered private practice, a common measure of "success" was the size of an office's support staff. There was no question that a large staff was a sign of a successful practice. **In today's competitive environment, more is not necessarily better**. A large staff is costly and often represents waste; however, small is not automatically better either. A small staff must combine the correct skill-mix, training and motivation to be maximally productive.

Simply cutting staff size in response to increasing costs or declining revenues can lead to lower quality. The quality that can suffer most when a staff is suddenly reduced is that of service (as measured by an increase in patient waiting time). This includes time spent waiting for an appointment, waiting in the reception room, waiting to schedule a procedure, or waiting for paperwork to be completed. How many HMO patients have come to your office and paid cash for necessary procedures because an HMO's wait time for scheduling a procedure was too long? This lower quality can trigger a downhill cycle, resulting in an inferior competitive position and lower profits.

Unfortunately, in an economic crisis, a business is forced to reduce staff size quickly. There is little time for thought about how to maintain quality while doing this. Fortunately, in spite of the negative possibilities, times of economic crisis offer an opportunity for improving quality *and* cutting costs. Staff can be reduced in ways which result both in a higher level of productivity and reduced waiting time.

There are three important considerations to be made when reducing staff size. The first is that one should never reduce staff without first reducing the number of staff activities. The second is that cross-training employees should be considered, since this reduces the number of people needed for a practice to remain fully productive during randomly occurring peak periods in either the front or back office. The third is that if employees are "empowered," an office becomes more effective.

Empowerment here refers to the transfer of authority and decision making from the doctor to the staff, the ones who are closest to operational problems and already have the information most relevant to handle them. All that is needed is additional training and the doctor's trust. Much has been written about empowerment in recent years, and it is important to understand the concept. The following observation should be helpful.

When I first started my practice, I listened to practice management experts speak on the topic, "Work Smarter, Not Harder." Practitioners tried to emulate these experts, and even with newly expanded staffs, many of the ideas learned from these experts were difficult to duplicate in their own offices. I feel one reason for this was that many of these "experts" had *special* staffs, not just *larger* ones. These staffs were special because a spouse often worked for the office. While one can argue the merits or demerits of a spouse working for an office, there is no question that a spouse is the ultimate empowered employee. Empowered employees are one reason that "mom and pop" businesses can operate with fewer employees.

It is important to understand that your staff can be this dedicated and productive too. Employee empowerment makes the difference. Imagine the efficiency increases possible if each employee had the same commitment to and knowledge of a practice that a spouse does. Everyone would be focused on what was best for the practice rather than on his or her individual job description. Empowerment does this. It is likely the "experts" didn't recognize that a major reason they had an easier time managing their busy practices was that they had at least one empowered employee.

A lot of books have been written about empowerment, but if you understand the above example, I believe that you already possess most of the knowledge required to begin empowering your staff. The easy part is instituting continuous training and teamwork. The difficult part is giving up control in order to gain commitment. Your effort will not be lost; there is less turnover when employees are empowered. **The combination of a reduction of activities, cross-training and empowerment becomes a powerful set of tools for achieving dramatic improvements in productivity with a much smaller staff**. In the future, higher profits and a superior competitive position will belong to those who can maintain a quality practice with the fewest number of committed employees.

The Funnel Process

Even when employees are fully trained and competent to perform a process, the outcome of that process will vary. The amount of variance is one measure of quality and is dependent on the design of the process. Individual employee skills are no longer the relevant issue in performance of a process. The process itself becomes the determining factor of performance and the predictability of outcomes. Yet, employees are often held responsible for events completely out of their control. **Poor quality is rarely attributable to an individual; it almost always indicates an inferior process design**.

An individual employee is powerless to change a process. Management is usually responsible for the design and control of processes, and only management is in a position to change them; however, optimum changes will occur within a process when there is participation by both management and all staff members responsible for the outcome of that process.

Consider the example of a simple "funnel process." An employee puts a marble into the top of a funnel, the marble rolls around the large opening until it reaches a small spout at the bottom of the funnel where it exits and falls into a target marked in a sandbox. A supervisor then marks and measures the exact impact point in the sand and records the measurement. The target is circular and has a "bull's-eye" at the center. The closer the employee gets to the center of the target, the higher the score and the higher the employee's pay.

At the end of the day, management compares scores and finds that some are above average and some below. Management then rewards the people achieving high scores with a bonus. While this may sound silly, it is precisely how most offices are run.

When we examine this funnel process, we find that the marble will land in different locations based on **random** statistical variation. It will never land precisely in the same spot twice. Statistical variation is the variation around a mean (average), and over time there should be an equal number of events on each side of that mean. In other words, by chance, there will be as many events above average as below. This type of variation is present in every process, is predictable and cannot be reduced without improving or changing the process.

Once an employee places a marble into the funnel, any outcome within the range of variance of the funnel is possible. The range of the variance is determined by the funnel's design, and any outcome within that variance range is considered to be acceptable quality. If the marble lands outside this statistically acceptable range, this outcome is related to something other than the process design (such as an employee mistake or mechanical problem). If an outcome is outside the acceptable range of variance, it is important to find and correct the cause. This **prevents** recurrences of problems, and prevention is always the least costly way of dealing with problems.

This funnel process could be any process within your office. If there is a problem with a process's output, it needs to be determined whether it is related to the process's design or to an extrinsic factor (such as inadequate employee training). If it is related to process design, the employee is powerless to do anything about it. If it is a problem unrelated to the process, it can be found and fixed with help from empowered employees. The majority of problems will be related to process design and not to employees. This type of problem can be corrected only if the doctor recognizes it as a process design problem and takes the necessary steps to improve that process.

Implementation of Change

Employee education, which includes cross-training, is a key ingredient for successful implementation of the efficiency concepts and ideas discussed in this book. When implementing changes of a larger magnitude, there will be a tendency for employees to resist or even actively sabotage the effort to change. While the primary purpose of this book is to teach business concepts, it is important to be aware of active or passive employee resistance because it can prevent the successful implementation of new ideas. Overcoming barriers to change and gaining employee trust are essential for successful implementation of change and will require employee participation. Two articles written by Kenneth Hultman, Ed.D., appear in the appendixes. These important behavioral topics are addressed in his articles.

CHAPTER

6

Understanding Processes and Technology

What Is a Process?

A process is a systematic series of activities or tasks directed toward some end. Everything that we do involves some type of process, including: getting ready for work in the morning, cooking a meal, or planning an evening out. The complete process of cooking a meal involves planning, shopping, cooking, setting the table, serving the food and cleaning up. Each process activity can be broken down into subtasks. For example, cleanup can be broken down into transporting dishes to the sink, removing waste, putting dishes in the dishwasher, sealing and storing leftovers and cleaning the table.

Considering that one of our goals is to reengineer office processes for the purposes of reducing cost, improving quality and increasing efficiency, I prefer the following definition of process: A process is any activity or group of activities that takes an input, adds value to it and provides an output to an internal or external customer.

We are all familiar with products produced by machines on assembly line manufacturing processes. The combination of reengineering and quality management techniques have led to dramatic efficiency changes for many of these manufacturers. These changes have resulted in cost reductions, increased productivity and higher-quality products. While these techniques work well for manufacturing processes, even greater overhead reduction can be achieved by applying these same techniques to business processes. Overhead costs created by inefficient business processes in a service business are a much higher percentage of those businesses' revenue than are the costs created for manufacturers by inefficient manufacturing processes. These costs to service businesses can be cut by as much as 40 percent through the creative application of manufacturing's reengineering and quality management techniques.

Business processes are a problem because they generally aren't "designed;" they "just happen" or result from an accumulation of "quick fixes" that develop in times of immediate need. They are never changed and, thus, become permanent. Each time a process is "fixed," additional activities or people are added to the process, and it becomes both more complicated and more costly. Processes are often a dependent series of activities (as in our example of the hike) that are activity oriented rather than outcome oriented. They are not customer-focused activities. This means that they contain costly statistical inefficiencies that increase cycle time. These processes are not only slow, they also have fundamental performance deficiencies.

Most businesses contain hundreds of processes and subprocesses. From the 80/20 rule, we can predict that 20 percent of these processes probably account for 80 percent of our cost and efficiency problems. We need to identify and understand these crucial processes first. It has been said that the best way to understand something is to attempt to change it. It is likely that if you ask everyone in an office to describe a process by drawing a flowchart of it, each one will draw a different diagram. This is a good place to begin.

Doctors often turn to automation with the hope of decreasing cost and improving the efficiency of their business offices. For many, automation has accomplished the opposite. It should seem obvious at this point that automation will not solve cost and efficiency problems without the processes first being redesigned. Automation should be applied to address specific problems such as bottlenecks, statistical fluctuations and wasted activities.

Enabler of Change

When new technology first arrives on the scene, it takes time to determine how it can best be used to make improvements. For example, when power surgical equipment was first made available, it did not significantly improve old surgical procedures. A modified McBride bunionectomy was basically the same whether manual or power equipment was used. If a doctor purchased a full set of power equipment only for the purpose of performing McBride procedures, it added cost to the procedure and was of little benefit. The real impact of power equipment was felt when creative thinkers were "enabled" by it to develop new and better procedures, ones that would not have been possible prior to the advent of this technology.

In this same sense, computers have enabled the development of new and better business processes. The problem is that when computers first became affordable for medical offices, many practitioners used them simply to automate old processes. This is analogous to using power equipment to "improve" the McBride procedure. Costs went up with no corresponding benefits. Just as in the example of power surgical equipment, opportunities do exist for computers to enable changes in business processes. They can be used in ways that make it possible for doctors to achieve the productivity gains and cost-reductions hoped for when they were first purchased.

Computers and Productivity

No matter what form health care ultimately takes, most physicians anticipate that they will be treating more patients at reduced reimbursement rates. In this price-competitive environment, two of the biggest challenges facing practitioners will be: 1) maintaining quality of care in the face of higher patient volumes; and 2) reducing or controlling office expenses that typically increase with higher patient volumes.

It seems logical to assume that computers, with their incredible speed and accuracy, might play a significant role in reducing overhead by enabling offices to become more efficient. A significant number of practitioners have already turned to computers for help. I assume that most of these doctors had hoped that office productivity would increase automatically with the use of computers and that this improved productivity would assist them in offsetting the impact of lower fees.

Unfortunately, in spite of rapid improvements in technology, few offices have successfully increased productivity or decreased overhead by using computers. Worse yet, many computerized offices have achieved exactly the opposite results.

Medicine's experience with computers is not unique. Service businesses have doubled their investments in computer technology during the last 10 years; yet productivity has grown only 0.1 percent a year in these businesses. In the early 1970s, Sears, Roebuck and Company believed that computerization would cut their costs by eliminating paper, the same belief that has been held by many medical offices. Instead, the amount of paper per employee went up 14,000 sheets a year with computerization.

Service-sector industries that have increased productivity by using computers are those that have been subjected to intense competition (e.g., the banking and airline industries). As competition in the health care industry escalates, increasing productivity becomes crucial for survival. If we are to achieve this with the aid of computers, we need to rethink their use.

In a 1991 paper, Stanford University economic historian Paul David compared the diffusion of computer technology to the replacement of steam engines by electric motors. With the first introduction of smaller, more efficient electric motors, industrial productivity actually decreased. David concluded that this was because factory managers used the first electric motors as substitute steam engines, much as the first computers have been used as substitute typewriters and adding machines. No positive impact on productivity was made by electric motors until factory managers realized that the principal advantage of a smaller and lighter engine was that it was easily portable. The electric motor could be transported to where the work was. After creatively rethinking the way these new machines could be used, productivity gains followed.

Many doctors still believe that office efficiency will improve automatically as computers become faster and software becomes more "user friendly." Speed and efficiency are both important factors when selecting a computer, but as was the case with the electric engine, a faster or more efficient computer will not, on its own, improve productivity. The computer must be used in a way that not only "speeds up" the process but actually changes and improves it.

A freeway commute in a car is a good comparison to the problem of whether to increase a computer's speed or to improve the process established for that computer. It takes an excessive amount of time to commute to work during the rush hour. If a 15-mile commute takes one hour during rush hour, will building a faster or more efficient automobile shorten the commute time? While a reliable car (which is capable of maximum freeway speeds) is essential, no further improvement in the car or its engine can effectively shorten this commute time. Shortening the time would require that the freeway system itself be redesigned (by such means as adding lanes) or traffic flow be improved (by such means as synchronizing traffic lights).

Productivity problems in our offices cannot be solved by fixing or improving machines either. Instead**, what is required is a change in the way we use those machines!** Redesigning our information flow (the highway system) and our work flow (the traffic flow) will produce the desired results.

Fortunately, our computer productivity problems differ from those of the automobile commute in that changing the "highway system" in a computerized office is not very costly and is under the doctor's direct control. Making these changes requires two decisions: 1) what are the changes that should be made; and 2) who should be responsible for making these changes?

To answer the second question: If our computer has a mechanical problem, calling in a hardware or software expert to fix the problem would be appropriate (just as a mechanic would be the right person to call to repair a car that is not functioning properly). If our goal, however, is to increase productivity through the use of a computer, technicians are not the experts who can help. The best "expert" for this task is you, the doctor. Each of our practices and situations is unique; therefore, our solutions will be unique.

Effective Computer Use

When medical offices first began to computerize, hardware and software costs were more than $25,000 for one computer! Because of this high cost, the first software processes developed for medical offices utilized only one computer that was located in the front office. Both technology and price have changed dramatically, but the business processes developed for use with our computers have not. For this reason, medical offices have yet to achieve a reduction in the cost of labor or an improvement in overall efficiency due to the introduction of computers.

Businesses tend to go through three distinct stages when converting from manual to computerized systems. During the first stage, there is little change. Work is simply done on an electronic screen rather than on paper. In the second stage, work speed is increased. When work is done both faster and better, the third stage is achieved. If medical offices hope to lower their costs without lowering quality, they must reach this third and final stage of computer usage.

Technology is not what holds us back; it is the way we use technology that does. In fact, most medical offices never complete stage one in their use of computers. Work is done on an electronic screen, but a complete backup paper process is also maintained. This is generally done because we are reluctant to trust new technologies. To maintain dual processes requires many wasted steps, more staff, and is therefore both more costly and less efficient than the manual system which has been "replaced."

Most doctors think that they are at least performing some work faster using the computer (our second computer stage). An illusion of speed exists because the computer is performing selected tasks much faster than was possible using the manual system; however, efficiency is not measured by the completion of any individual task. Rather, it is measured by the completion of a **group** of tasks forming a process designed to produce a finished product or service; i.e., the total cycle time of the process.

While some individual tasks might be completed faster using a computer, the entire process is not. One reason for this is that the computer process links both slower and faster tasks together in a series of interdependent steps requiring the completion of one task before the next can be started. The process is not finished until all process tasks are completed, as was the case in our example of *The Hike*. The hike was not completed until the last scout arrived at his destination. The slowest task in the process functions as a "bottleneck," just as our slowest hiker was the bottleneck for the scout troop. It is important to identify the bottleneck because it is at this point that the speed and efficiency of the entire process is controlled.

To better understand the effect bottlenecks have on efficiency, it is helpful to return to the example of the freeway. Any bottleneck might be a fixed one (such as when three freeway lanes narrow to two) or a randomly occurring one (such as an automobile accident that temporarily closes a lane at a random point along the freeway). If a bottleneck on a freeway lengthens a commute by an hour, any improvement in the speed or efficiency of the cars on that freeway will not lessen the total commute time. Such an "improvement" would simply allow cars to rush faster to the bottleneck point where they would then sit and wait for their turn to pass through. The greatest efficiency measures for improving the commute time would be developed by focusing on locating and improving the bottleneck point. "Speeding up" any other component of this commute would be a waste of time, effort and money.

The traditional way to "fix" a bottleneck is to remove it or find a way to go around it. Freeway engineers solve such structural bottlenecks by adding lanes or by changing the direction of the flow of traffic at selected times. The location of random bottlenecks cannot be predicted in advance; they can only be addressed by such tactics as removing a damaged vehicle as quickly as possible while redirecting traffic flow around the vehicle before and during removal. Fortunately, there are easier and less costly methods for dealing with randomly occurring bottlenecks in business processes.

The best solution for any bottleneck would be to instantly add one or more lanes around it. While such a solution is not possible with freeways, it is possible with office computer processes. Parallel electronic "lanes" for computer processes can be created by adding remote terminals networked to a central system; however, simply adding remote terminals and networking computers does not automatically address a bottleneck. The network must also employ processes designed to utilize these additional lanes. These lanes can then be used to increase capacity at bottlenecks or to bypass them.

Bottlenecks create a need for additional employees, and they lower the quality of service by increasing cycle time. "Fixing" them will create a significant decrease in total overhead costs, improve quality and achieve the desired third stage of computer use where work is done both faster and better. Competing successfully in a managed care environment will be easier if your computer is used at this most effective stage.

CHAPTER

7

Business Process Improvement and Reengineering

Why Process Improvement?

Dr. W. Edwards Deming, the quality guru of manufacturing processes, estimated that, "Most troubles and most possibilities for improvement add up to proportions something like 94 percent that belong to the system and 6 percent to special causes." The "system" in a medical office is the collection of business processes, and "special causes" include such things as employee mistakes and equipment breakdowns. If 94 percent of troubles belong to the system, the majority of our efforts should focus on process improvement. This is the most effective way to make progress in cutting costs or increasing efficiency.

Office business processes are what drive both the cost and quality of a service business. When we improve processes, we generate more profit and increase competitiveness by focusing on customer needs. In fact, improving or redesigning business processes will increase profit more than anything else you can do.

Business processes have a great deal to do with a patient's perception of quality of care. Manufacturing companies have determined that a customer is five times more likely to turn away because of a poor business process than a poor product. I know that every time I take my car in for servicing, I swear I will never buy a car of the same make again. I can put up with mechanical breakdowns, but the service quality of the repair shop is often more than I can tolerate. There is no question that I would buy the same car again if I were happy with the service.

The same perception of quality is true for medical offices. Excessive time spent in waiting rooms, mistakes in billing, failure to call with important lab results and appointment errors are all service problems that can lead a patient to believe that the quality of medical care may also be low. This is usually more than a perception. The problems created by poor business processes are distracting and time consuming for doctors. This time would be better spent in patient care. Patient complaints regarding difficulty in accessing an office can also lead a PPO or an HMO to "delist" a doctor.

Expediting

Manufacturing companies usually employ people who function as "expediters." If a customer is upset about an overdue order and calls to complain, an expediter will go through the shop, find the status of the order and determine what is holding it up. Invariably, he or she finds the order in line with others, waiting for a process task that can only be performed by one machine, the bottleneck machine.

The expediter will move that order ahead of the others and follow it through the shop to completion. The customer is then called and given the good news that the problem has been handled and the order is on its way. What about other customers, waiting patiently, who haven't called to complain? It is likely that the next time they need to reorder, they will quietly go somewhere else.

Most employees who work in a business know how to expedite an important order or service. To accomplish this, they need to "go around" the process. They simplify and speed up the process by "cutting through red tape." If a process is so inefficient that everyone knows how to go around it, maybe the process itself is bad and should be redesigned. Expediting is a key symptom which signals that a process should be improved, and the method that people use to go around a process often gives the first clue as to how it can be fixed.

Existing Processes

Most of a medical office's existing business processes are put together with little thought. When a doctor first begins a practice, he or she has few patients, and little need exists for processes capable of handling a high volume of patients, phone calls, or paperwork. Process improvement is driven by practice growth that continually places strains on different processes at different times. Process improvement becomes a series of "putting out fires." If the phone becomes too busy, an additional person is hired to help answer it. If paperwork falls behind, a computer is purchased and more people are hired to input data.

As an office or clinic grows, the processes become more complicated, more costly and less efficient. Many are designed as dependent series, similar to a series set of holiday lights. Each process change simply adds one more bulb in the series instead of converting the process to a parallel one. In spite of the money spent in "adding bulbs," the overall process is not improved.

Many processes become rife with wasted activities, bottlenecks and large statistical fluctuations as a practice grows. Customer focus is lost, and the changes made are no different than adding highway lanes in front of bottlenecks or raising the speed limit on a congested freeway. Some activities that are not wasteful are added to processes, but they add no value for the customers.

The processes become long, cumbersome, bureaucratic and difficult to manage. Each "process fix" is essentially a Band-Aid necessary for immediate repair, and over time, the process becomes an accumulation of Band-Aids and quick fixes with little thought as to how each addition will affect the whole. In the "old days," the higher cost of inefficient processes made little difference in profitability. Today, however, it is a different story.

While managed care has its positive side, the negative impact of declining fees, higher patient volumes and increasingly complex paperwork is magnified by the high cost of inefficient business processes. For this reason, increasing the efficiency of business processes can be critical for success in a managed care environment. A list of the important business processes encountered in the typical medical practice can be found in Appendix Three.

Scope of Change

Process improvement is employed when a process is a good one but needs to be made better. Process reengineering is used when the process has been ineffective and needs to be redesigned. When an incremental process change is needed (one of 10 percent or less), process improvement can be utilized, but if a 30 percent, or greater, change is desired, reengineering is necessary. There is a large "grey area" in between where combinations of the two will work, improving some processes while reengineering others. There are similarities in the methods of process improvement and reengineering, but there are important differences, and the decision of which method to use should be made ahead of time.

The key difference between process reengineering and process improvement is that a totally new process (process reengineering) cannot be created by simply making incremental improvements (process improvement). Often, radical change requires designing a new process from scratch. As an example, no matter how much time or money is invested improving a propeller engine, the effort will never result in a jet. The jet engine can only "happen" by starting over with an entirely new concept (jet propulsion) and "reengineering" from scratch. While there are environments appropriate for either type of engine, the best and most improved version of a propeller engine cannot compete with the "worst" jet if speed is the critical factor for success.

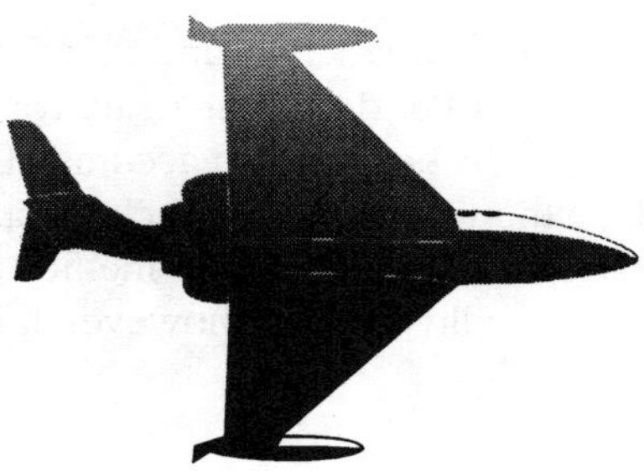

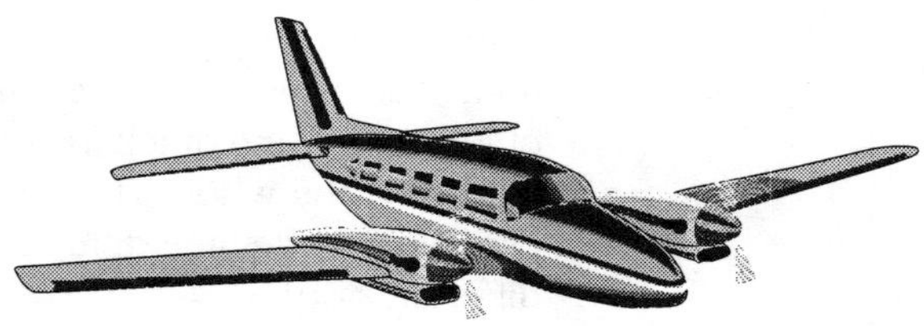

Process improvement is less disruptive than reengineering, but the return (as measured by both profit and efficiency) will be correspondingly less; however, the more skilled and creative the doctor is at using concepts presented in earlier chapters, the more benefit can be achieved from process improvements. Process improvement is faster and can accomplish a great deal with little capital. Because of the speed of implementation and low requirement for capital, a process can sometimes be effectively improved first and then reengineered at a later date.

Process improvement begins with the identification and selection of key processes that might benefit from improvement (The Pareto Graph, or *80/20 Rule*, might be used here). One should focus first on those processes with the potential of providing the biggest "bang for the buck." The processes selected should be critical to customer satisfaction and have sufficient opportunity for reducing the types of problems that lead to higher costs. In the example of making a propeller plane fly faster, the improvement team would first identify the "critical success factors" for speed. In this case, the improvement team might decide to focus on the propeller engine, the weight of the plane and the design of the wings. If this were a medical office, the team might choose to focus on the processes for insurance billing, medical records and patient scheduling.

Business Process Improvement requires an initial investment of time to understand the existing processes. BPI begins with each person who works within a process drawing a flowchart of the process. Each flowchart represents one individual's understanding of how that process "works." This is an important exercise because each person understands the process in a different way, and all the flowcharts may be different. The procedure of diagramming a process immediately begins to identify problems and stimulate thinking for potential solutions.

This procedure of drawing and comparing flowcharts is continued until each person understands the process in the same way and agrees that one final chart accurately reflects the existing process. This exercise will also identify process participants who may have been inadvertently excluded from the process improvement team. It is possible, too, that the process "team" may be only one person.

Improvement is directed at **simplifying** and **streamlining** the process. This is accomplished by analyzing flowcharts based on the existing process and finding opportunities for the following changes:

1) eliminating bureaucracy (empowering and cross-training employees);
2) reducing cycle time (eliminating bottlenecks and wasted activities);
3) eliminating activities that add no value from the customer's perspective;
4) eliminating activities that add more cost than value;
5) reducing interruptions;
6) eliminating duplication;
7) converting series to parallel activities;
8) standardizing tasks;
9) reducing processing time; and
10) reducing task variances.

After analyzing an existing process, the team should evaluate improvement ideas and "quantify" them in terms of cost, time saved, money saved, or customers helped. If a financial investment is needed, it should be determined whether the final benefit (the bottom line) is greater than the investment. **We already know by definition that if bottlenecks or wasted activities are eliminated, a process automatically will be more efficient, less costly and more customer focused**. Often these changes are costless, but if they involve purchasing technology or hiring more people, an accurate quantification and comparison needs to be made between the cost of the changes and the expected benefits.

Before implementing any new ideas, the "improved" process flowchart should be diagrammed and inspected for additional improvement opportunities. The flowchart serves as a low-cost "model" for testing the new process.

Once implemented, the improved process should be continuously improved. This can be accomplished through periodic meetings scheduled to discuss the process and by looking for ways of streamlining even further using the 10 categories of change listed above. This becomes a search for bottlenecks. Remember that whenever a primary bottleneck is eliminated, the next slowest activity becomes the new primary bottleneck. Bottlenecks will be easier to spot after wasted and non-value-added activities are eliminated, and the constant focus on eliminating or speeding up bottleneck tasks will continuously improve a process.

Automation

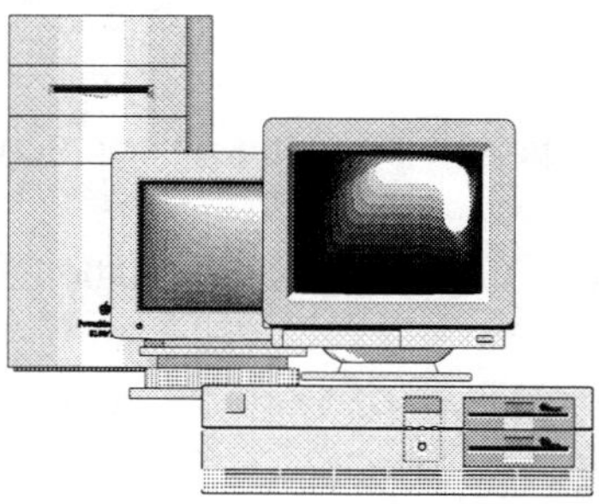

Specific suggestions for the use of automation in addressing critical medical office business processes will be covered later under reengineering. Unlike reengineering, business process improvement methods reserve the use of technology until after a process has been improved. It is easier to automate a streamlined process, and the process team will have a better idea of the benefits they hope to achieve from automation. If medical offices improve their processes first, it saves the practitioner headaches and the added complexity that occurs when automating cumbersome and inefficient existing processes.

If an improved process is to be automated, the computer should be used only to further reduce or eliminate bottlenecks and wasted activities. Otherwise, it will not improve the process and could actually make it worse by hiding problems.

Eighty percent of most process activities are repetitive and could benefit from automation; however, computerizing a process simply to speed up repetitive tasks, such as printing insurance forms, might be premature. This may prevent a computerized process that goes well beyond simple improvement from being developed. Some critical processes have interrelationships which allow them to be integrated into a single new process, to be redesigned (reengineered) from scratch. This requires more analysis and planning, but the payoff can be substantial.

Reengineering

Future profitability, and perhaps even survival, of a medical practice is largely dependent on lowering costs and increasing productivity. Despite the fact that we now have less control over fees and volume, we will always have control over costs and productivity. This same problem has been dealt with successfully by other competitive industries. Other industries have been forced to develop better tools for dealing with these problems to remain profitable. The challenge now is to adapt the successful tools they have developed to the specific needs of medicine.

"Reengineering helps us solve that modern business dilemma—how to do more with less and do it better," said Ronald E. Compton, Aetna chairman (in the June 14, 1993, issue of *Business Week*). He was referring to the application of new tools designed to radically change critical business processes with a resultant dramatic cut in overhead and improvement in quality. There are no quick, easy or painless solutions to cost and efficiency problems, and reengineering is probably the most disruptive method of all; however, for those who remain persistent, the rewards of reengineering are well worth the effort. Overhead in a service business can be as high as 80 percent of costs and could possibly be cut by as much as 50 percent with reengineering.

The Total Quality Management technique of Continuous Quality Improvement is highly effective for improvement of business processes that are fundamentally sound. Unfortunately, most of our business processes are not fundamentally sound because they were not carefully "designed." As mentioned before, they either just "happened" or resulted as an accumulation of "quick fixes" developed to meet immediate needs. Fixing these processes requires radical change using reengineering methods rather than incremental change using Continuous Quality Improvement methods.

While computers enable the reengineering process, simply purchasing new hardware and software will not change a process for the better. Many doctors have attempted to address cost and efficiency problems by investing in the latest technology. Unfortunately, most have automated their **existing business processes** rather than first improving or reengineering these processes. Because of this, these doctors' experiences have been similar to those of most other service businesses that have done the same: costs went up, and efficiency went down. H. James Harrington, author of *Business Process Improvement*, summarized this point well with the following statement: "Automating a bad process not only ensures that we can do a bad job every time but that we can do it faster and with less effort than before."

To reengineer a process, we need to sit down with a blank sheet of paper and redesign the process from scratch. Because reengineering can be disruptive to an office, not all processes should be redesigned at once. Begin with the most critical (costly) ones; it is here that the potential savings are greatest. Focus on creative ways to achieve the desired outcome from the process. For example, the desired outcome of accounts receivable management is to get paid for our services, not to age and track receivables. Some offices waste time focusing on individual process steps, such as aging and tracking, rather than on solving the question of why the receivables became "old" in the first place. Remember, a shorter and faster process is easier and less costly to manage, requires fewer employees and achieves the desired outcome both sooner and more often.

Several years ago, my office went through the upheaval created by reengineering critical processes. The most significant "discovery" we made in the area of computerization was that **the type of hardware and software used was far less important than the physical location of the computer in the work flow**. For example, in our office, the relatively "simple" process of rescheduling patients involved 14 steps, and the receptionist was frequently interrupted while scheduling patients over the phone. Computerized schedules located in the reception area did not change the process because they simply performed the traditional process with the substitution of an electronic screen for paper. The work flow was exactly the same; however, moving computerized scheduling to the back office changed everything dramatically. This process change was not a simple change of location; it dramatically changed the scheduling process for the better. The process had been reengineered.

With this change in our process, the number of steps required for scheduling went from 14 to two, and all four potential patient waiting periods (bottlenecks) were eliminated. Costs decreased because scheduling time was reduced by six minutes per patient. In addition, productivity increased because multiple personnel were now able to schedule appointments simultaneously during random peak telephone periods. Our quality increased because back-office personnel were able to schedule our time more effectively than a receptionist in the front could. These back-office personnel estimate future time requirements for a patient more precisely. This enables them to place patients in "better" time slots (less waiting time), and the receptionist is no longer interrupted during patient phone calls (fewer patients put on hold). The "nuts and bolts" of reengineering the scheduling process will be discussed in more detail in the next chapter.

As we tackle each business process, our results are the same. I am convinced that the winners in the future health care delivery system will be those who are able to successfully reengineer their critical business processes, thus gaining a significant competitive cost and quality advantage. There is no other method that can improve cost and efficiency more dramatically. Most importantly, the cost improvements gained through reengineering are more permanent than those achieved through "quick-fixes" that often lower quality.

Waiting Time, Cycle Time and Customers

Efficiency can be defined in many ways. The most useful definition (one that can lead to better decisions) is: efficiency is a comparison of the value of total output to the total cost of input.

Any investment or effort designed to improve efficiency must either raise the quality (value) of service as perceived by the customer, lower the cost of overhead, or both. There are numerous places where one might seem to be improving efficiency within a process without lowering costs or adding value. Under our definition, this type of efficiency is waste. The challenge is to identify those areas where one can add more value than cost to a total operation.

Richard J. Schonberger, author of *Building a Chain of Customers*, states, "If there was one single measure of quality, especially quality of service, waiting time (or lack of it) is probably it." For purposes of our discussion, waiting time will include the time intervals between all activities of a process, whether we are looking at clinical procedures, scheduling or paper processing.

Americans value quick service. Because of this, a reduction in waiting time will increase the value of a service to the customer. The correction of problems that lengthen waiting time often leads to simplification of processes, and simplification reduces errors, lowers costs and builds a significant competitive advantage as a byproduct. The search for opportunities to reduce waiting time is not easy, but at this point, you already understand the basic concepts needed to begin.

The concepts of throughput time and cycle time are important in management. In manufacturing, cycle time is used to define the time interval between completed units. Throughput time is the time necessary for one unit to go through an entire system. These concepts apply equally well to patient treatment and paperwork processing in a medical office or clinic. It is important to note at this point that in the service industries, **reducing cycle time has come to mean reducing both cycle and throughput time.**

For example, a medical office might have an average throughput time of 75 minutes per patient and an average cycle time of 10 minutes. This means that the average patient would spend 75 minutes in the office, and one patient would exit the office every 10 minutes (six patients an hour). It is financially important for the doctor to treat at least six patients an hour, but for the patient, it is important that the 75-minute throughput time not increase.

It was discussed earlier how the cycle time for the entire process in a multistep operation is determined by the cycle time of the slowest step in that process. Understanding this point is necessary for quality improvement and cost-reduction. Reducing cycle time alone allows additional volume to be processed (good for the doctor), but it does not reduce waiting time, which would be good for the patient, and therefore it adds no value for the patient. The slowest step of a process acts as a bottleneck for that process, and eliminating a bottleneck will shorten both the throughput and the cycle time. Therefore, with a focus on eliminating bottlenecks, both the doctor and the patient benefit because total waiting time, costs and productivity will all be improved.

When I discuss the reduction of cycle time throughout the remainder of this book, assume that this means the reduction of both cycle time and throughput time. This will be true because our focus on the elimination of bottlenecks and wasted activities will automatically reduce both.

It is important to remember that increasing speed in a non-bottleneck location only adds cost. Such a change will not reduce cycle time; it only serves to increase the number of patients (or size of the stack of paper) waiting at the bottleneck. Practices routinely invest money "improving" non-bottleneck activities with the hope that the entire process will improve.

Bottlenecks are not easily recognized in a busy office; however, a skillful use of ongoing training in the topics covered in this book and the proper use of teamwork can facilitate the discovery of their locations. To utilize teamwork effectively, it is helpful to redefine the term "customer."

We all understand that the patient is our final customer; however, each person in a medical office or clinic has another customer, and that customer is the person in the work team waiting next in line to receive his or her work. Improving the quality of service to each "next customer" ultimately will improve the quality of service to our final customer, the patient. Drawing a process flowchart will help to identify the relevant internal and external "customers."

Under managed care, the term "customer" includes not only those mentioned above but also managed care organizations, referring doctors and employers. With an oversupply of providers, these customers can be selective. I believe that the better an office is able to deliver cost-effective, efficient, quality care, the more demand there will be for its services. Efficiency increases the value of an office's services relative to competitors. While cost is currently the principal focus of health care reform, the long-term goal of large corporations is to purchase value. Businesses understand that the current attention is on the direct cost of health care, but they also know that the indirect costs, such as wage replacement and lost productivity, can average four times more than direct costs.

I believe that the best strategy for physicians facing a cost-competitive medical environment is to survive over the short term while positioning their practice to thrive over the long term by delivering value. Ellen Gaucher of University of Michigan Hospitals defines value as, "a combination of outstanding clinical quality, outstanding service quality and cost effectiveness. **Health care systems must focus on the improvement of all three**." Efficiency improvement through reengineering is the only way to improve all three simultaneously!

In a multi-employee office, process reengineering begins with the formation of teams that include staff members working within the process selected for improvement. Because a team would include all relevant "customers," and it would be searching for bottlenecks and wasted activities, the solutions it finds will be focused on the most important concerns, customer concerns, and we have learned that when work teams become "customer focused," they, by definition, become "cycle time focused."

Some processes only need improvement while others need to be reengineered. Most reengineering efforts will be unique for each office. Office layout, number of employees, type of software used, location of equipment and many other features will be different; however, there are generic conditions that will be similar for all offices. These will be considered next.

When a process is reengineered, several jobs are usually combined into one. This is the way an office functions when it is starting out. Private practitioners often start with one employee, and this employee knows every job in the office. Later, as the practice grows and employees are added, each employee becomes more specialized and is less able to perform other duties. When this concept was discussed earlier, it was in the context of demonstrating how cross-training and empowerment can help improve productivity during randomly occurring peak periods and eliminate the need for additional hiring. One important reengineering technique is similar to this, combining several jobs within the same process into one. If sequential tasks in a process are performed by the same person, the problem of "accumulation of slowness" from statistical fluctuations is reduced, and cycle time is improved.

An office or clinic needs to be reorganized around processes rather than tasks. When several jobs are combined into one, there are opportunities in offices and clinics for one person to manage a complete process. If one person is in charge of a process, there is less chance for customer focus to be lost.

Another positive feature of reengineering is that office staff members are involved in the decision making. This is one of the goals of empowerment. Empowerment works best when it is used in the context of reengineering. By "works best," I mean that the employee not only enjoys his or her job, but when he or she makes decisions, they are the type that improve customer satisfaction and profit.

Another aspect of reengineering is that of "hybrid centralized-decentralized operations." Later, we will be discussing a "hybrid" version of centralization. A model for merging medical business offices will be presented. This model presents the example of combining business operations while retaining separate clinical practices. This, or any other type of practice merger, will lower costs **only** if business processes are reengineered first.

Decentralization is important in large corporations for reducing the number of managers. In order to successfully decentralize, empowerment of employees is essential. Decentralized decision making is better because it places decision making in the hands of the people with the most relevant information for making those decisions. This is important for your medical practice, too.

The final concept to be discussed at this time is that, when reengineering, work should be performed "where it makes the most sense." For this purpose, reengineering frequently involves changing the physical location of office equipment. Computer technology now allows us opportunities to overcome many physical barriers that were previously quite formidable, if not impossible to change (e.g., the simultaneous availability of charts in multiple locations). This concept and its application to computerized scheduling is discussed in detail in the next chapter.

CHAPTER

8

Reengineering the Scheduling Process

In addition to achieving a lower-cost position, competing in a managed care environment will require the capability of managing and treating a larger volume of patients effectively. To this end, efficient scheduling is a tool that can help to build a competitive advantage.

I recall many days when my appointment schedule appeared to be overbooked, yet I ran on time and finished on time. I also recall other days when the schedule didn't appear to be "busy," yet I ran behind all day while somehow finishing on time. It appeared to me that there were many times when patients didn't arrive in the right order. Also, patients were often scheduled for inappropriate amounts of treatment time.

In the service business of medicine, the "product" that we "sell" is our time. It makes sense that our overall efficiency (and profitability) is dependent on how well we manage that time. The standard tool used by doctors to manage time is the appointment book. If we hope to improve efficiency and compete in a managed care environment, we will need to "rethink" this tool and how it is used.

Approximately two-thirds of today's practitioners have converted to a "computerized office," yet only a small percentage use their computers for managing patient appointments. Many practitioners initially utilized their computers for patient scheduling but later discontinued this use because they had experienced no improvement over their old paper appointment books. I have read several articles where "experts" concluded that computerized scheduling was inefficient.

The reason that most practitioners experienced no efficiency gains with computerized scheduling was that they had simply substituted electronic screens for paper appointment books. The work flow had remained exactly as before. The only change was that scheduling appointments had become more complicated because additional training was now required to perform the "same old job."

CASE TWO: PATIENT SCHEDULING

At the end of a busy day, Dr. Jones was informed by his receptionist that she needed help answering the phone and scheduling patient appointments. She stated that she could handle the calls most of the time but that there were several hours during the day when she had too many people waiting on hold, and she would lose calls. She also noted that during these busy periods, some patients who were waiting to schedule appointments on their way out of the office became annoyed because of the wait and left without rescheduling. Even the people she was able to speak with had to be rushed off the phone, and this left them with a poor impression of the office. In addition, she was unable to greet arriving patients in a timely manner.

Dr. Jones told the receptionist that he would investigate the problem but added that he could not afford to hire additional help. On the following day, he announced that the front-office staff was to begin assisting the receptionist in making appointments during peak phone periods. One week later, he was informed by the receptionist that nothing had changed. When other front-office staff answered the phone, patients were simply asked to hold and wait for the receptionist to pick up the phone and schedule appointments. When the doctor asked why these patients were put on hold, he was informed that there was only one appointment book, and for this reason, only one appointment could be scheduled at a time, regardless of how many people answered the phone. The same thing happened to patients exiting the office who wished to be rescheduled.

In addition to these problems, Dr. Jones was frustrated because the schedule never seemed to "flow" well. Some patients were booked for too much time and others for too little. This often resulted in rushing new patient exams, which left these patients with a poor impression. He wondered why this happened and how it was possible for him to run behind all day and still finish on time.

Dr. Jones purchased a computer and installed an electronic scheduling system with the hope that this would solve some of his scheduling problems. After everyone had learned the new system, the paper appointment book was replaced by the computer. After implementing the new process, nothing seemed to improve. In fact, the staff felt that the problem had worsened. The electronic schedule took longer to learn, and unlike the paper appointment book, it could not be moved to another location in order to schedule an appointment.

The "final straw" occurred when Dr. Jones was interrupted in a treatment room in order to receive a call from a patient. He determined that the patient needed to schedule a minor procedure. He put her on hold and left his patient in the treatment room while he went to the front office to discuss the caller's future appointment with the receptionist. Despite the fact that the receptionist was on the phone with another patient at the time and two other patients were waiting in line to schedule return appointments, Dr. Jones asked her to take this call ahead of those waiting patients.

As the doctor returned to the treatment room, one of the patients waiting in line for a return appointment became irate and announced that it was not fair that the patient on the phone had been assisted ahead of her. She left the office without rescheduling. When the doctor returned to the treatment room, he had to spend an additional few minutes explaining to his patient waiting there why it had taken him so long to return.

Before hiring an additional receptionist, Dr. Jones decided to read *Reengineering the Medical Practice*. When he returned to the office, he immediately began to attack his scheduling problem by examining the work flow and collecting data that he felt was relevant to solving these problems.

Optimizing the Scheduling Process

When Dr. Jones analyzed his scheduling process, he found that a significant bottleneck occurred as exiting patients arrived at the front desk to schedule a return appointment. The same individual who answered the phone and greeted arriving patients also made appointments for exiting patients. In this three-doctor office, multiple patients often exited at the same time, and as they lined up at the front desk, they were frequently ignored by the receptionist who was occupied scheduling a "phone-in" appointment.

This bottleneck created several problems: 1) exiting patients waited too long for appointments at the front desk; 2) at the same time, phone calls were being put on hold; and 3) patients received inappropriate appointment time (either too much or too little) because the receptionist was rushed and did not always know exactly what treatment was to be done on the patient's next visit or how long it would take. Dr. Jones was frustrated that other employees were unable to help with this bottleneck even though they often had free time and possessed the information necessary to schedule most of these appointments.

After drawing and analyzing numerous flowcharts, the office staff realized that their existing process was a dependent series of steps with numerous wasted activities. Dr. Jones knew that the best way to "fix" a series process was to convert it to a parallel one. Instead of hiring a new staff person, he changed the office work flow by adding "parallel lanes" to this process. A computer network, with terminals at multiple locations, was installed and enabled the office to accomplish this task.

With a terminal located in each treatment room, appointments can now be made by either the doctor or the nurse before the patient leaves the treatment room. The exiting patients are able to bypass the front desk, and if the phone is "ringing off the hook," cross-trained employees are able to help answer it and schedule appointments from multiple locations. The need for an additional employee in the front office has been eliminated, and the receptionist has even gained slack time, allowing her to help in the back office during peak treatment periods.

The chart below compares the before and after scheduling cycle time:

	Before	**After**
Discuss return visit with the doctor	2 min.	2 min.
Mark and transport routing slip	30 sec.	0 min.
Average wait at the front desk	3 min.	0 min.
Discuss return visit with receptionist	2 min.	0 min.
Discuss appointment options	30 sec.	30 sec.
Book appointment	1 min.	30 sec.
Additional conversation with busy receptionist	1 min.	0 min.
Total time	**10 min.**	**3 min.**

The first step in this new process is for the doctor to discuss the return appointment with the patient. This is "quality time" between the doctor and patient and adds value. This step remains identical in duration to what it had been in the old process. Except for scheduling the appointment, each remaining step is wasted "cycle time" that adds no value for the patient. The new process retains the "quality time" and reduces the remaining cycle time. In a high-volume office, this excessive cycle time had translated into a great deal of wasted time and aggravation for both patients and staff.

The time savings of this new process would be reason enough to switch to electronic scheduling; however, even greater gains were achieved from the improved quality of the schedule and patient flow that occurred as a result of the change. The doctors have become more involved in the scheduling process, but it takes them no more time than before, and doctors are the ones who have the most to gain from the improved patient flow. When patients are seen in a more efficient order, they are happier and don't waste valuable treatment time complaining about how long they had to wait in the reception room or giving the doctor suggestions about how to run the office.

Dr. Jones's original intent had been simply to reduce pressure on the receptionist and eliminate the need for an additional employee; however, the quality of his schedule improved dramatically and benefited the office in more ways than he had anticipated. This occurred because doctors and back-office nurses have the most in-depth knowledge of the requirements of return patients and are, therefore, able to schedule patients most effectively. The resultant effect has been that the practice is able to run on time more consistently despite a significant increase in patient volume. This new process is both less costly and more effective than the old one.

Another benefit of electronic scheduling can be seen when the doctor is interrupted to take a call from a patient. If an appointment is needed for the patient, the doctor can now schedule it during the telephone conversation. This avoids the wasted time that occurs for both the doctor and the receptionist when the receptionist needs to be interrupted in order for the nature of an appointment to be explained. It also enables the doctor to make the decision as to where to "work this patient in," which is especially important when the schedule appears to be "full."

The next chart depicts the advantage of a doctor being able to schedule a patient over the phone when he or she is interrupted in a treatment room.

	Before	After
Phone interruption	0 sec.	0 sec.
Dr. travels to phone	30 sec.	30 sec.
Average conversation time	2 min.	2 min.
Dr. walks to front desk	30 sec.	0 sec.
Wait for receptionist	30 sec.	30 sec.
Talk to receptionist	30 sec.	0 min.
Receptionist discusses appointment with patient	2 min.	0 min.
Book appointment	30 sec.	30 sec.
Additional conversation with receptionist	30 sec.	0 sec.
Total Time	**7 min.**	**3 min.**

The doctor is not removed from the treatment room, and the calling patient is able to receive an appointment scheduled for the appropriate amount of time.

If any additional evidence is needed regarding the benefits of scheduling from the treatment room, the system can be compared to an alternative used by a clinic with which I am familiar. This clinic used centralized scheduling. It often ran three hours behind schedule; yet it finished on time at the end of the day! This was clearly a work-flow problem caused by patients arriving in the wrong order and receiving an inappropriate amount (too much or too little) of scheduled treatment time. The clinic was manned by a renowned group of doctors who were supported by a large staff. In spite of this "high quality," its high cost and poor service (who wants to wait three hours?) was a prescription for failure, and it ultimately closed.

A person who does scheduling in a centralized scheduling situation has the least amount of information needed to make an optimum patient appointment. A receptionist located at an individual clinic has better information, but the doctors and nurses working with the patient have the "best" information of all. This is why hospital operating rooms run behind schedule even though they schedule twice as much time as most offices do for the same procedure when done in-office. The current lower cost of computer technology affords us the opportunity to adapt electronic scheduling to a more effective and efficient use.

Scheduling Flowchart 1 (page 128) demonstrates Dr. Jones's original scheduling process. This process is long and complicated and has many unnecessary "waits." Each wait provides opportunities for patients to either hang up or leave without making an appointment. This flowchart demonstrates an inefficient and costly process with a high degree of variance during busy periods, and in spite of its high cost, this system produces a poor quality schedule.

Scheduling Flowchart 2 (page 129) demonstrates an attempt to "improve" the process by using a computer. From this flowchart, one can easily see that this computerized process is the same as the old one. The work flow is unchanged, and all bottleneck and wasted activities are still in place. ***Scheduling Flowchart 2*** **demonstrates clearly why computerization has neither improved efficiency nor cut costs for many medical offices**.

Compare both processes with the reengineered process depicted in *Scheduling Flowchart 3* (page 130). It can be seen at a glance that this new process is simpler. The new configuration of the computer network has changed the work flow and enabled the following: 1) elimination of fixed bottlenecks (by converting a series process to a parallel one); 2) elimination of randomly occurring "peak period" bottlenecks (by allowing cross-trained individuals to simultaneously schedule appointments from any location); 3) elimination of unnecessary activities and their associated statistical fluctuations; and 4) elimination of the need for more employees. In addition, this streamlined and lower-cost process also produces a higher-quality schedule.

SCHEDULING FLOWCHART 1

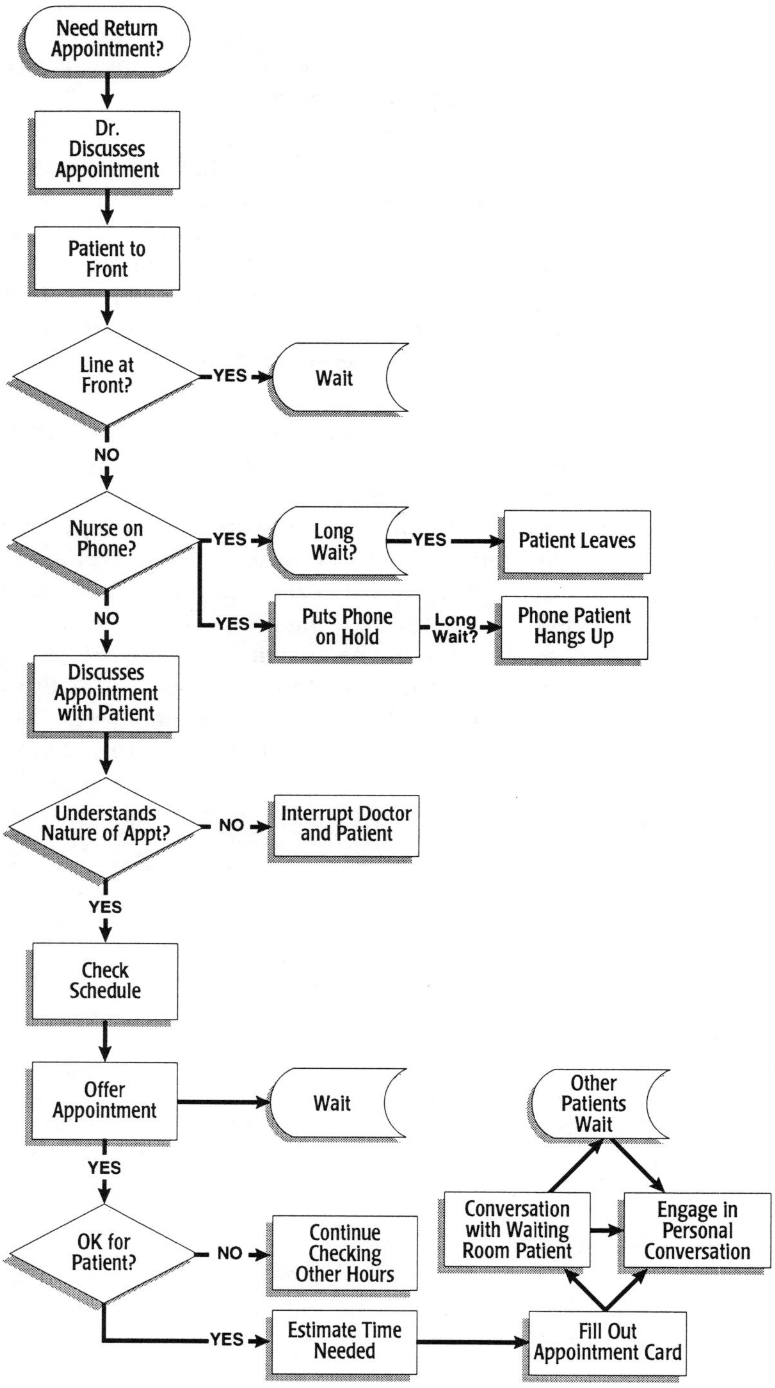

SCHEDULING FLOWCHART 2
ADDING A COMPUTER

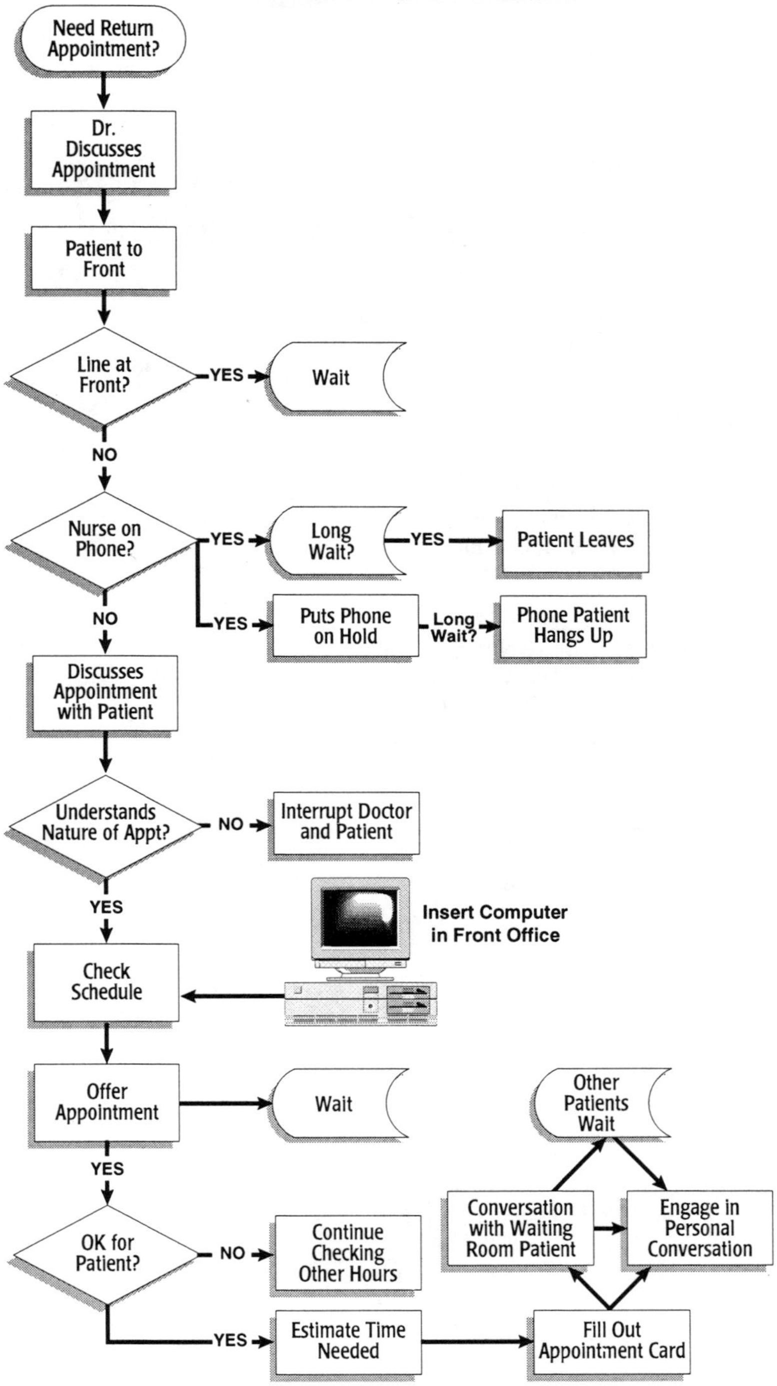

SCHEDULING FLOWCHART 3 (REENGINEERED PROCESS)

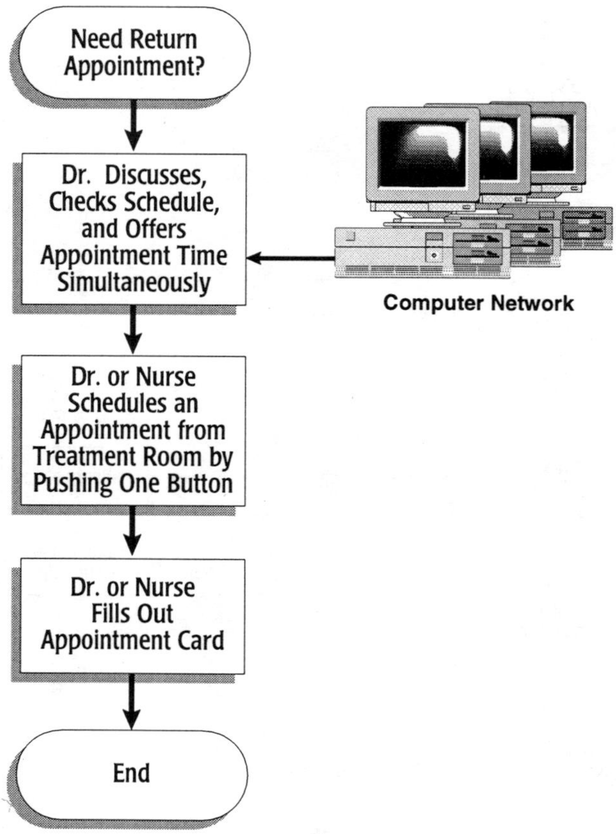

CHAPTER

9

Reengineering the Billing Process

CASE THREE: DATA ENTRY

Dr. Jones was pleased with the progress he had made cutting costs and improving his quality of service to patients. Now that his scheduling process had been improved with no additional personnel, he was ready to attack his billing process. The office's collection ratio had dropped from 80 percent to 70 percent, and he felt that this was a result of inefficiencies created by higher patient volume and increasingly complex insurance billing. He calculated that if he could restore this ratio to 80 percent, his collections would increase from $1,000,000 to $1,142,856. When his billing staff approached him to request additional personnel to help them "catch up" on the insurance billing, he knew it was time to act.

Dr. Jones began to analyze his billing process the next day. Data were collected, and a flowchart was made. He was surprised by a long delay at the point where superbill data were entered into the computer. His staff responded that it was more "efficient" to accumulate several days of data to enter all at one time. Just as with his scheduling problem, he was frustrated by the inability of personnel with slack time to help "speed up" the billing cycle. Again, he could not afford to hire additional staff.

What options were open to him? **Are there options that might improve the process and reduce the need for more personnel at the same time?**

Data Entry and Billing Process Efficiency

As we have seen, every service a doctor provides is accomplished by completing a series of interrelated tasks, which combine to form a distinct process. Medical offices use numerous business and treatment processes, each designed to deliver a specific service. As practice revenues continue to decline under managed care, the most effective response is to reduce overhead expenses by streamlining these costly processes.

In the "scheduling example," it can be seen how the bottleneck activity controlled the efficiency (and hence the cost and quality) of that entire process. Similarly, a cost-cutting and improvement effort for the billing process needs to focus on finding and "fixing" bottleneck activities.

Data entry is one of many tasks within the billing process. It happens to be the first activity in the process, one that must be completed before the rest of the process can proceed to its goal (which is to collect money). While bottlenecks can be located anywhere within a process, the entry of data into the billing process is a bottleneck activity located right at the beginning of the process. Let us focus on opportunities for eliminating this particular bottleneck, with the expected result of reducing the cost of billing and increasing the collection percentage of an office or clinic.

Most medical offices utilize a paper superbill for the purpose of recording a patient's diagnosis and services performed on any given visit. This superbill is attached to the patient's chart, and the doctor marks it after he or she has completed the necessary patient care. The superbill is then transported back to the front office where the data it contains are entered into the computer.

What happens after superbills arrive at the front office? Most often, they are accumulated in a large batch, as they were in Dr. Jones's office, and the data are entered later, often on the following day (or even later if an employee is absent). One difficulty caused by this delay is that no other component of the billing process can proceed until this initial data entry has been completed.

There are two significant problems with this process: 1) it is functioning on an inefficient, one-lane highway; and 2) it requires tasks that add no value to the outcome of the billing process. Fixing this data entry bottleneck should improve the efficiency for the entire billing process and free up valuable employee time for more productive activities.

As was shown previously, the best way to fix bottlenecks is to either remove or go around them. **In this case, we can do both.** We can go around the bottleneck by adding one or more "electronic lanes," and we can eliminate the use of paper superbills altogether. Both of these goals can be accomplished by adding remote computer terminals in the treatment rooms, putting superbills on the computer monitor and networking these terminals to the front office. Now, rather than marking paper superbills, the doctor can enter the identical data (only faster) onto his or her electronic screen. To see the efficiency benefits of this new process, it is helpful to compare it to the old one.

The old process entailed printing a superbill, recording the patient's name and account number on that superbill, attaching it to the chart, transporting it to the treatment room, marking the diagnosis and treatment, transporting it back to the front office, adding it to the batch of superbills waiting for data entry into the computer and finally filing this superbill in the patient's chart. Even with all of these tasks being performed, no information is available in the computer regarding the patient's charges or his or her contracted financial responsibility when that patient is ready to exit the office. This results in the probability that the office will either collect no money at the time of the visit or overcollect on the visit, requiring that a bill or a refund be sent to the patient at a later time.

In contrast, the new process is always current, even when front-office employees are absent. Rather than marking a paper superbill, the doctor enters the identical data directly into the computer from the treatment room. This takes him or her less time than it had previously taken to mark a paper superbill. **Every other process step discussed above is eliminated.** Now, when the patient exits the treatment room, any available employee (including the doctor) can check the computer screen and instantly see what portion of the total bill is the patient's responsibility. If desired, that correct amount can be collected on the day of the visit. This is especially important under contract medicine and Medicare because these balances are often small, and the preparation and mailing of thousands of invoices or refund checks is costly both in time and supplies.

Most software programs have the capability of automatically making contractual deductions and adjusting a patient's balance to reflect correct fees and adjustments for Medicare or any other of the many insurance contracts you may have. This is done at the time that data from the patient's visit are entered. The balance can then be collected at the time of the visit so that when the insurance check arrives, the ledger is automatically adjusted to zero. No bills or refund checks need to be sent.

In our office, having the doctors enter data directly into the computer in the treatment room had the immediate effect of eliminating one full-time position. In addition, the shortened billing cycle made it possible for the remaining employees to focus on accounts receivable at a point much earlier in the billing cycle. This resulted in a 10 percent improvement in our collection ratio. This higher collection ratio, combined with a reduction in salaries, helped us to counter the negative impact on practice income caused by lower fees.

Submitting claims electronically presents yet another opportunity to shorten the billing cycle and improve the collection ratio. Eliminating the tasks of printing and mailing insurance forms provides more time for collecting overdue accounts.

Perhaps the most important advantage of our reengineered billing process is still to be realized. If survival under managed care necessitates that we treat a significantly higher volume of patients, we should now be able to manage the corresponding increase in paperwork without adding employees or working overtime.

The following chart compares "before" and "after" cycle times achieved from reengineering the work flow and moving data entry from the business office to the point of service. The time savings are considerable, and there is no longer an overnight (or longer) storage time. The doctor is spending no more time than before, and if he or she had previously transported the superbill to the front office, that doctor now spends less time completing this process. Prior to reengineering, when a chart was refiled before a copy of the superbill was filed in it, the time of filing and refiling the chart would need to be added to the "before" column of our chart. The opportunity for such large variances to occur in the "before" processing times is highly likely, and the size of these variances is not accounted for in the total times indicated below.

	Before	**After**
Mark diagnosis	10 sec.	10 sec.
Mark treatment	15 sec.	15 sec.
Transport	20 sec.	0 sec.
Overnight storage	24 hrs or more	no
Data entry	60 sec.	0 sec.
File in chart	10 sec.	0 sec.
Total	**24 hrs 115 sec.**	**25 sec.**

It is interesting to note that the original process would be considered highly efficient by most medical billing standards. The data were usually entered the day following treatment, and insurance forms were generated and mailed (or electronically transmitted) within a few days following data entry. Special causes, such as an absent employee or a physician's delay in marking the superbill, could create large variances and delay the process. I am aware of some clinics where physicians might delay marking a superbill for several weeks or longer, resulting in a lower collection ratio and lost charges. This problem is avoided with electronic superbills because charges are done "on the spot," and we are never behind.

On the following page are "Data Entry" flowcharts, comparing the data entry process before and after reengineering. The original "computerized" data entry process is on the left. It can be seen that this process work flow is basically the same whether or not the computer is used. The computerized process is the same as the old paper process with the exception that the need to spend extra time balancing a day sheet is eliminated in the "computerized" version.

Compare this with the *After Reengineering* chart on the right side of the page which depicts a shorter and more streamlined data entry process. It can easily be seen that the process work flow is dramatically different when the computer is inserted at this new point within the process.

DATA ENTRY

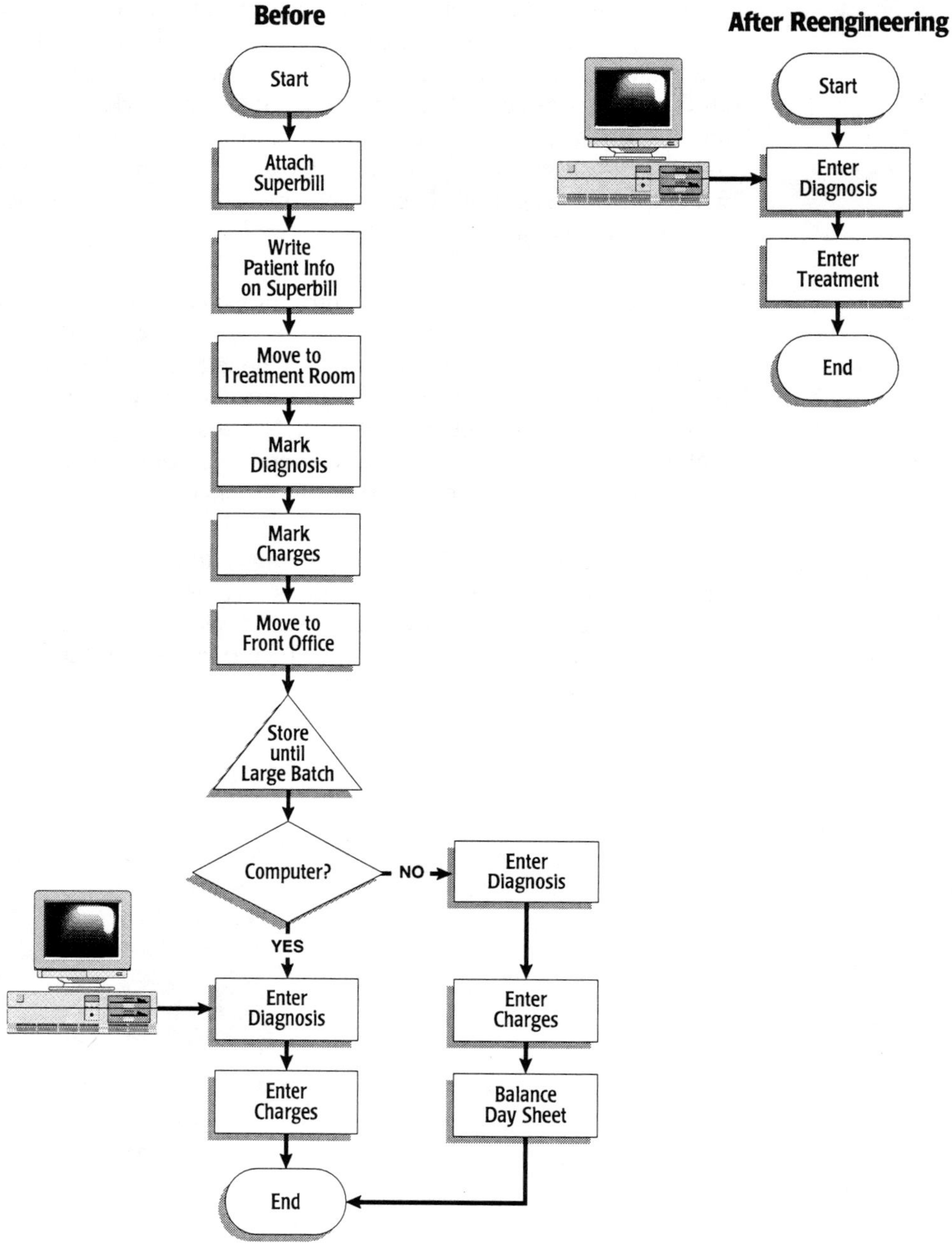
Before
Start
Attach Superbill
Write Patient Info on Superbill
Move to Treatment Room
Mark Diagnosis
Mark Charges
Move to Front Office
Store until Large Batch
Computer?
NO
Enter Diagnosis
Enter Charges
Balance Day Sheet
YES
Enter Diagnosis
Enter Charges
End
After Reengineering
Start
Enter Diagnosis
Enter Treatment
End

CHAPTER

10

Reengineering the Charting Process

CASE FOUR: THE CHARTING PROCESS

One evening Dr. Jones was completing the chart of a diabetic patient who visited the office every two months for a relatively minor preventative treatment. The patient had been coming to the office for eight years, and this patient's diagnosis and treatment were always the same. When the doctor completed the chart, he decided to refile it rather than leave it for the staff to file the next day. When he attempted to return the chart he was actually unable to fit it back into the file cabinet. He wondered, "Why is this chart so thick?"

The doctor began to look through the chart and found superbills, insurance forms, several reports for minor procedures and written notes that were mostly identical for each visit. He then wondered, "How much time does it take to put all this in the chart? Does it need to be there?" When he posed these questions to the staff the following day, they said that they felt it necessary to file a copy of everything, even though the exact same information was already stored in the computer, because there was a possibility that the computer would "crash." When the doctor asked if the filing was time consuming, they responded that filing was not a problem because the office had hired a full-time person to do that job!

After further analysis, Dr. Jones collected data and drew a flowchart of the charting process. He was amazed at the number of complicated movement and filing process steps each chart went through. The only place where value was added to the chart was when notes were written in it by the doctor, and 80 percent of the time, these notes were virtually carbon copies of the previous visit or were of routine postoperative visits. He also noted that many of the notes (especially those written by one particular doctor) were almost illegible. Might there be a solution that would improve this process and reduce the number of employees at the same time?

Automating Medical Records

Most hospitals are actively investigating methods for automating patient records. The typical problems associated with hospital records include illegible handwriting, time wasted locating the one copy of a patient's chart, or looking through hundreds of pages in a chart for answers to questions. In addition to solving these typical problems, computerization allows the introduction of innovative methods for expanding the patient record to perform new functions, such as: coordinating patient information to support clinical decision making, alerting physicians to adverse drug reactions and providing management with information needed for broader strategic decisions regarding competition under managed care.

While there are many details that still need to be settled before determining the best method for automating medical records, it is important that the efficiency principles described in earlier chapters not be ignored when considering computerization of office medical records. While it is easy to see that computerization can improve the quality and function of medical records, the current plans of most hospitals ignore efficiency considerations and, because of this, their utilization of computers will ultimately increase rather than decrease the cost of the medical records process.

Many doctors are either using or contemplating the purchase of software designed to automate the charting process. As we have learned, automation does not necessarily make an existing process better or less costly. Do you recall Sears's attempt to eliminate paper by computerizing? Instead of eliminating it, automation actually increased the volume of paper per employee by 14,000 sheets a year. While this is one possible outcome if medical record automation is not managed properly, opportunities do exist to improve the efficiency of charting systems when technology is applied in a manner that eliminates wasted activities and increases the speed of bottleneck activities.

It was estimated in *The Wall Street Journal,* April 6, 1992, that the cost of managing paper records in medicine is at least $5 per patient visit. Dr. Albert Martin, president and chief executive of InterPractice Systems, maintains that an electronic chart will save as much as $10 a visit. This dollar savings comes from reducing waste (such as eliminating unnecessary activities), eliminating paper backup systems, reducing storage, increasing the speed of finding and searching charts and eliminating filing. As a result, quality is better because charts are immediately available, more legible and more complete.

Electronic charts offer other advantages in addition to money savings. Consider that in a typical hospital, 38 percent of a physician's time is spent charting patient records, and 30 percent of the time charts are not even available to the doctor at the time of patient treatment. These "unavailable" charts are either misplaced, in transport, or in use elsewhere at the same time. A typical chart weighs 1.5 pounds, and this means that my office alone creates more than one ton of paper charts a year, all of which must be stored!

The following example depicts some of the steps utilized by offices for managing charts: Charts are pulled the evening before appointments, moved to the front desk, opened and have treatment sheets inserted, stamped with the date, transported to treatment rooms on the following day, reviewed by the doctor (with notations made or dictated), transported back to the front office, and filed back "in place." Additional steps are created later when retrieving the chart to file **unnecessary** papers into it, including copies of superbills and insurance forms which are already stored in the computer.

How might a computer be used to improve this process? In the above example, the only **necessary** step is the one in which the chart is being used in the treatment room to review previous treatment or to record notes. To improve this process (i.e., lower the cost while making it better), the computer can be used to eliminate unnecessary chart movement and filing steps, and reduce the time doctors or nurses take to dictate or make notations in the chart; however, most doctors are accomplishing none of this with their automated charting processes.

Consider the following example of a doctor who was touting a new computer software program he was using, whereby charting was done with a scanner and bar codes. This doctor stated that his system had made charting more efficient. When asked what occurred after he entered data into the computer, he stated that the information was then printed on adhesive paper, cut into strips and pasted into charts. I wondered, "How is this more efficient? This process retains all the old wasted steps, and it adds even more by requiring the subsequent retrieval of charts, cutting and pasting, and refiling of charts." In my office, this "improved" process would require that we hire an additional person.

One might argue that this system would reduce the amount of time required of the doctor for making chart notations. This is certainly possible and should be one of the main goals of automation, but what about staff time? Why print out the notes? This system would be more efficient if the notes were retained in the electronic form and paper charts were eliminated altogether. A computerized process that retains all charting information in an electronic form will eliminate every chart movement and filing step while providing the doctor the opportunity to further reduce his or her charting time by automating routine notes. Notes can always be printed out when they are needed for a specific, **productive** purpose.

While automating medical records can result in significant improvements in office efficiency, the greatest efficiency gains will be achieved by integrating charting with other processes. **On a typical day, the average patient visit generates at least 10 wasted charting steps, eight wasted data entry steps and six wasted rescheduling steps.** Eliminating these unnecessary activities reduces the total number of steps in these three processes from 29 to five. The doctor's focus can now be directed toward finding additional creative methods for using the computer to reduce the time required to complete the five remaining steps. This is especially important because these five steps are all steps performed by the doctor.

Following our office's successful integration of electronic scheduling and data entry, we were able to reduce our staff size by 40 percent without sacrificing quality. We have streamlined our charting process but have not yet eliminated paper charts. We do not anticipate that fully computerizing the charting process will eliminate any additional employees, but it will provide both the doctors and remaining employees with time that can be used more productively. Another benefit of the new process is that if we increase patient volume, we will not require more employees to manage the corresponding increase in paperwork.

The following table compares our predicted "before" and "after" cycle time necessary for managing one chart. Note that with the exception of the process step "writing in the chart," every other process activity is waste and can be eliminated. The only way cycle time can be reduced further is to automate and reduce the processing time required for making chart notes.

	Before	After
Retrieve charts	45 sec.	0 sec.
Open and date	10 sec.	0 sec.
Insert new sheet	10 sec.	0 sec.
Move chart to back office	10 sec.	0 sec.
Write in chart	75 sec.	75 sec.
Move chart to front office	10 sec.	0 sec.
Storage (file charts later)	yes	no
File "things" in chart	30 sec.	0 sec.
File the chart	45 sec.	0 sec.
Total	**235 sec.**	**75 sec.**

The flowcharts below and on the following two pages demonstrate the charting process. *Flowchart 1* demonstrates the original charting process and *Flowchart 2* illustrates the "computerized" charting process. Again, note that the computer did not change the work flow. This is essentially the same process. The computer may actually even add steps. *Flowchart 3* is the reengineered version of our process. Note that the work flow has now been significantly changed with a dramatic reduction in the number of process steps.

CHARTING - FLOWCHART 1

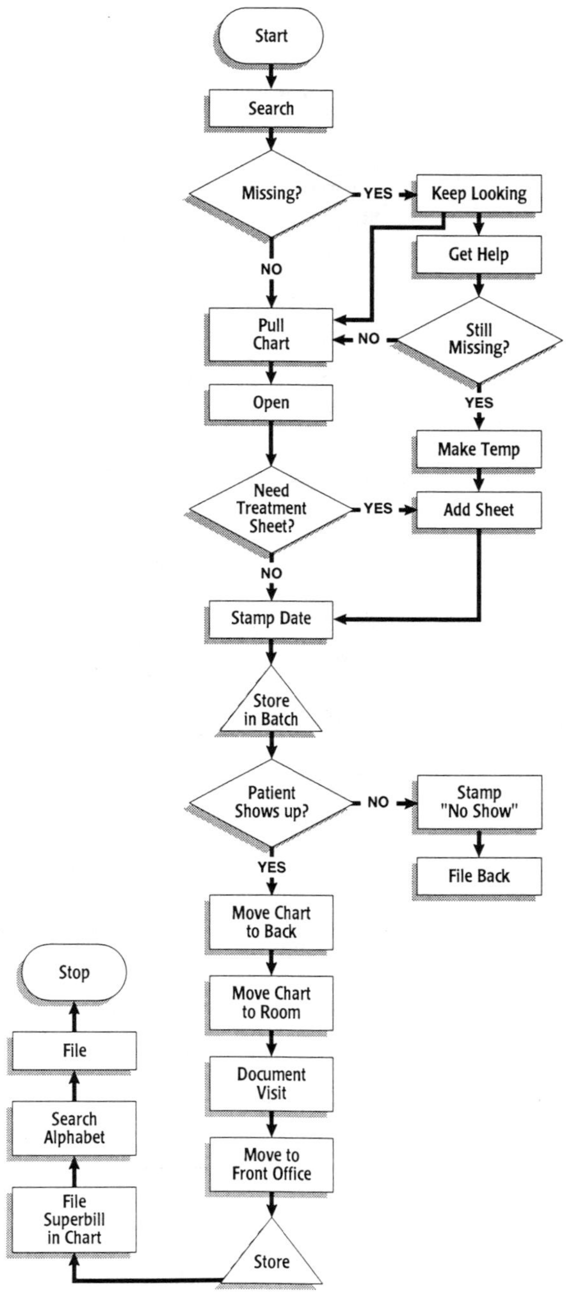

CHARTING - FLOWCHART 2

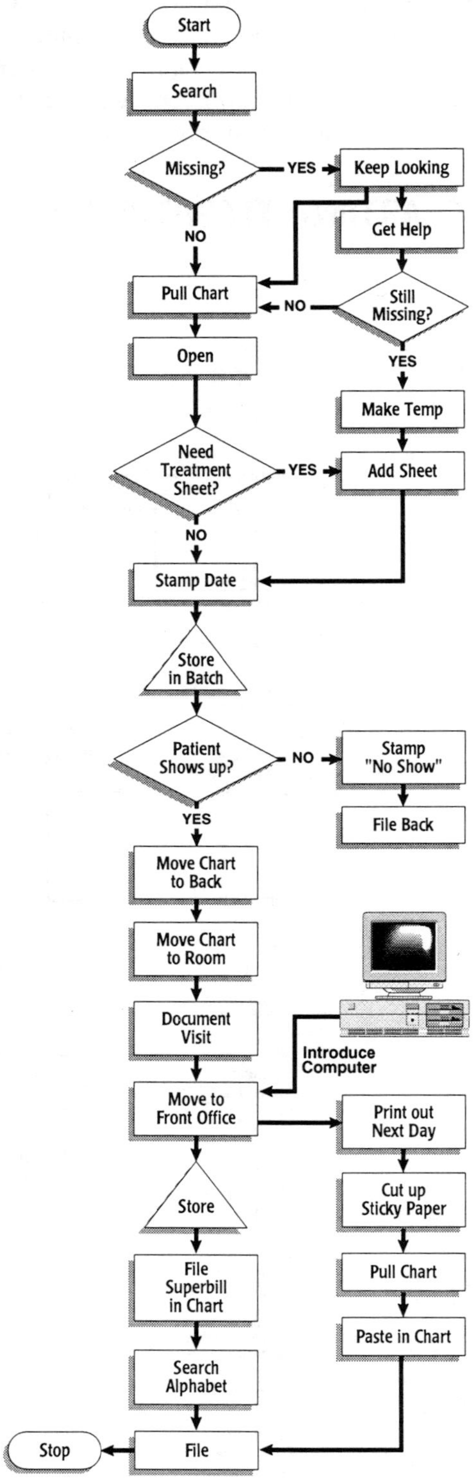

CHARTING - FLOWCHART 3

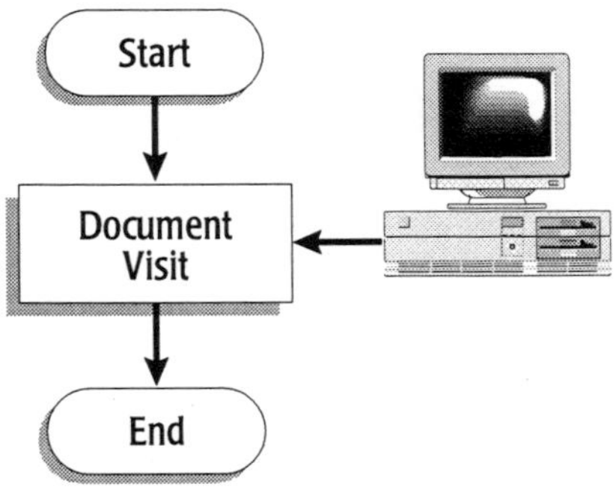

It can be seen that the charting process here has been reduced to one activity. It is clear from this flowchart that any further improvement of this process must focus on reducing the processing time required to document a visit. At this stage, improving the software process is the focus, and it should begin by drawing new flowcharts and looking for bottlenecks and wasted activities. Some of the necessary changes may require working with the software manufacturer. With software innovations such as the use of scanners, bar codes, voice recognition, and touch-screen data entry, the future possibilities for reducing charting cycle time are limited only by the doctor's and the computer programmer's imaginations.

Cost Benefit

Integrating multiple business processes in this way requires having a computer terminal in every treatment room, especially if electronic charting is one of the processes to be used. To determine the cost and benefit of such a purchase, consider that a five-treatment-room practice would require one main server and five networked terminals. If it costs $2,000 for the server, $6,000 for five terminals ($1,200 each) and $5,000 for software and accessories, the grand total would be $13,000. If this amount is financed at 9.5 percent, the monthly payments would be $273. Compare this with the potential savings in salaries, the improved quality of the processes and the ability to manage growing volumes of patients and paperwork in a more cost-effective manner.

CHAPTER

11

Communication and Work Flow

Communication Efficiency

To function successfully, all businesses need to develop efficient processes for the communication of information. In the past, large businesses "solved" internal communication problems by adding costly layers of middle managers who functioned as information messengers between the top and bottom levels of an organization. Over the years, price competition has forced many companies to rethink this method and look at less costly and more efficient ways of facilitating communication.

Much of the "downsizing" that businesses have found essential to survive in competitive environments has been accomplished through the elimination of middle-management positions. Computers have accelerated this process by facilitating the flow of information throughout organizations and thereby making many middle-management positions redundant. Smaller businesses, such as medical practices, have more recently begun using computers to assist them in this downsizing process.

There are different levels of urgency for receiving diverse types of information. Some is needed quickly and must be communicated before it would be available in a computer database. For this reason, it is often necessary for both large and small businesses to continue to employ people who function primarily to relay urgent information. Smaller businesses, however, can utilize methods of communicating quickly that are not readily adaptable to larger businesses, methods that sometimes eliminate the need for "middlemen."

Several years ago, an "essential" back-office employee left our practice. Her leaving had an immediate negative impact on back-office efficiency. In spite of this, we were slow to begin looking for a replacement for her position. During the time that we were functioning "shorthanded," we noticed that the greatest impact on the office caused by this employee's absence was the loss of ability to quickly communicate specific information necessary for follow-up patient care. In reality, a significant amount of this nurse's time had been spent functioning as a middle manager.

The type of "middle management" that this nurse had been providing is demonstrated in the following example: Assume that the doctor is interviewing a new patient while two other patients are waiting in treatment rooms. The doctor determines that x-ray films of the new patient are needed; however, before he is able to begin treating another patient, he must first locate a nurse, interrupt her from her routine, explain which x-ray views are required (and on which patient) and then inquire as to the location of his next patient. This results in **both** the doctor and the nurse being unable to perform productive work during this exchange of information. Previously, our "extra" nurse would have performed this liaison function.

A meeting was convened to discuss this problem. During the meeting, several other office communication problems were recognized and a list was developed. The list included the following questions: 1) How might the doctor communicate follow-up patient care information (x-ray views, procedure set-up, redressing, etc.) to the back-office nurse without spending time looking for or interrupting her? 2) How might each doctor in this group practice easily be able to determine for himself which patient he is to see next? 3) How might the front-office assistant be able to easily recognize which room is available for a patient entering from the waiting room?

As various alternatives for communicating this type of information were discussed, most were eliminated because they were either too slow, too costly, or required that we hire an additional employee to implement them. The nurses suggested a "visual" system. This system was to consist of plastic "flags" that would make information available to all employees at a glance. This seemed workable because it was inexpensive, quick, and the office had been designed so that all treatment rooms were visible from any location within the office.

The system that our office staff developed consists of sets of six different colored small plastic flags, costing $32.75 per room, at a total cost of $294.75 for our nine treatment rooms. The flags are mounted outside our treatment room doors using Velcro so that they can be removed easily if anything needs alteration. In our office, the flags are distributed as follows: 1) Three of the flag colors are allocated to the doctors. Each doctor is assigned his own color in order to know which patients are his, where they are located and how many are waiting for him; 2) A fourth color flag signals that x-ray films are needed for the patient in that room (the nurse can check the chart in the room to see exactly what angle and view are required); 3) A fifth color signals that a procedure is to be performed on that patient (again, the nurse can check the chart to see which set-up, consent, anesthetic, etc., is needed); 4) The sixth color signals that the patient needs some type of follow-up care or that the room needs to be cleaned; 5) All flags down indicates that the room is clean, empty and available for the next patient.

These flags provide a significant amount of information at a glance. When a doctor needs assistance, he writes the necessary information in the chart, displays the appropriate flags, exits the room, scans the treatment room flags for the next waiting patient and goes to that room. This system has eliminated many unnecessary interruptions and has saved valuable time for both doctors and nurses, time that is better utilized for direct patient care.

In addition to improving intra-office communication, the use of a visual flag system has resulted in the elimination of one full-time, back-office position. This, combined with our prior elimination of two front-office positions (which resulted from reengineering the billing and scheduling systems) has produced a 40 percent reduction in our staff size. In spite of this reduction in personnel, patients now receive appointments sooner than they did before, and once they are in the office, they spend less total time in the office (less cycle time).

The flowcharts on the following page compare our old communication process with the new one. The new process is less complicated and was inexpensive to implement.

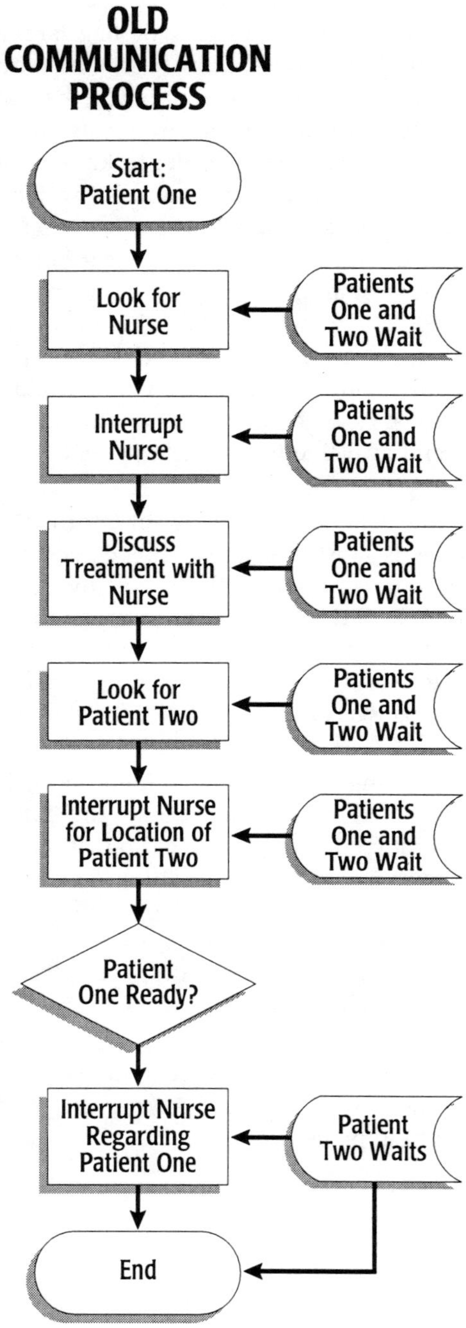
OLD COMMUNICATION PROCESS
Start: Patient One
Look for Nurse
Patients One and Two Wait
Interrupt Nurse
Patients One and Two Wait
Discuss Treatment with Nurse
Patients One and Two Wait
Look for Patient Two
Patients One and Two Wait
Interrupt Nurse for Location of Patient Two
Patients One and Two Wait
Patient One Ready?
Interrupt Nurse Regarding Patient One
Patient Two Waits
End

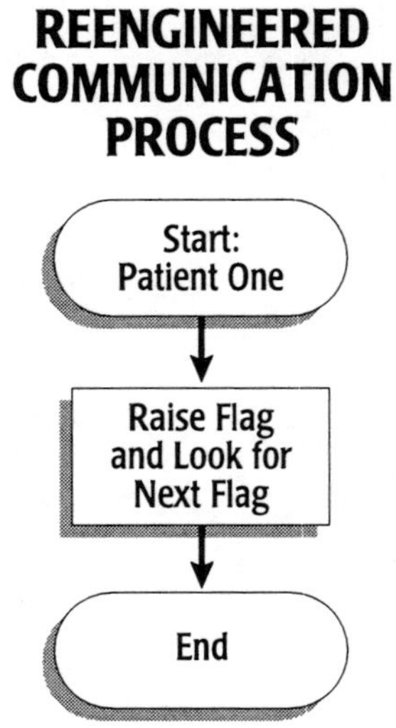
REENGINEERED COMMUNICATION PROCESS
Start: Patient One
Raise Flag and Look for Next Flag
End

CHAPTER

12

Finance

Understanding Pricing Dynamics and Discounted Contracts

With the emergence of a variety of new reimbursement methods under managed care, it has become apparent to business entrepreneurs that doctors have neither a basic understanding of fees nor a rationale by which to set fees. It is no wonder that physicians frequently ask, "How do I evaluate a contract if I can't determine whether or not the reimbursement rate is acceptable?" I can guarantee that if a doctor does not understand the dynamics of how his or her current fees were determined, that doctor will be at a disadvantage when faced with determining which new contracts will be acceptable.

It was stated in *Harvard Business Review*, September 1992, that "Getting the price right is one of the most fundamental and important management functions; it should be one of a manager's first responsibilities, a nuts and bolts kind of job that determines the dollar and cents performance of the company." Business people know that doctors have a weakness in this area, a weakness that many have no hesitation exploiting.

The first time I realized I did not understand the complexities involved in pricing was during the gas shortage of the 1970s. At the height of the gas "shortage," I remember hearing an economist say that when the price of gas reached $1.25 a gallon, the lines at gasoline stations would disappear. I wondered, "How can he predict that?" Do you know what? He was right! His calculation was actually a relatively simple one based on knowledge of the **elasticity of demand**, in this case, the demand of gasoline. Elasticity is one example of the many interrelated concepts that come into play when making pricing decisions.

In the past, physicians were able to function easily without understanding pricing concepts because medicine was not a highly competitive industry and demand was relatively inelastic. In that environment, physicians could raise fees whenever their profit margins fell and only create a minimal reduction in patient volume. As soon as medicine became a competitive industry, plagued with an oversupply of physicians and an overcapacity of hospital services, it began to fit the same model as other highly competitive industries. The old strategy of raising fees to compensate for declining profit margins was no longer viable.

Before discussing the concepts involved in pricing, let us first see how fees should **not** be determined. Fees should not be determined by: 1) a doctor's overhead (cost plus mark-up); 2) other physicians' fees; 3) what a doctor needs to earn; or 4) what is "fair." Unfortunately, these are methods traditionally used by many physicians.

There are three interrelated levels of price management in a competitive marketplace. The first is industry supply and demand, and this includes the concept of elasticity of demand. The second is market strategy. This addresses the areas of the service package that patients and third-party payers perceive as important, and attempts to determine the amount they are willing to pay for superior service. This is where market research tools come into play. The third is transactions. This is the most important level to understand before accepting discounted contracts. Understanding the difference between average cost (the cost your accountant typically gives you) and marginal cost (the actual cost of accepting new business) is critical to understand this level of pricing.

The dynamics of pricing in medicine are more complicated than those at play in the gas shortage example. This is because medicine offers many services, and the demand for its services is influenced by third-party payers. There are, however, other industries that have both multiple services and third-party payers (the defense industry, for example), and for all these industries, basic pricing concepts are the same. The main difference between medicine and other industries is that most other industries are managed by people who understand the dynamics of pricing and its effect on demand in their own industries.

Physicians almost always concede pricing responsibility to business and finance people, leaving doctors at a disadvantage when it comes to evaluating contract risk. A more level playing field could be achieved if practitioners possessed the same basic pricing skills and knowledge as businessmen and women. These skills and knowledge could be applied by practitioners to decision making regarding the contracts on which they want to bid.

It is important to understand the difference between "optimum" and "maximum" when discussing pricing. It should be our goal to treat the optimum number of patients, not the maximum. When a business moves past "optimum," and its volume approaches maximum capacity, it becomes less efficient and less profitable. No factory operates regularly at maximum capacity, and in our practices we also must optimize volume if we wish to maximize profit. Every practice has its own optimum mix of patient volume and types of service. The strategy of many practitioners is to continue to add patient volume at any fee. This strategy is flawed and, in the end, not sustainable.

The Relationships Among Price, Volume and Revenue

Even with improved efficiency, a practice will have difficulty surviving if its pricing and volume are suboptimal. A practitioner must answer two critical questions before making any pricing decision. The first is, "What is the optimum fee I can charge for each service to maximize my profit?" The second is, "If a contract sets a fee below my optimum, what is the lowest contract or service fee that I can accept and still make a reasonable profit?"

The answer to these questions will be different for every practitioner because each practice has a different cost structure and elasticity of demand. This is why copying the fees of other doctors or accepting all contracts available are not correct strategies. We will focus first on the question of how to maximize revenue and, following this, we will focus on evaluating discounted contracts.

Most of us understand intuitively that volume and price move in opposite directions. As physicians' fees increase, demand for their service tends to decrease (experienced as a drop in patient volume). In reverse, a fee decrease should increase patient volume. The problem is that most physicians assume that maximizing either fees or patient volume will lead to higher revenue. This may not be the case. Instead, **the goal should be to maximize total revenue by *optimizing* fees and patient volume rather than *maximizing* them.**

Remember that revenue is the product of price and volume ($R = P \times V$). When you raise prices, the law of supply and demand predicts that volume will go down. The relevant question is: Does revenue go up or down? It could go in either direction; the result is dependent on the **price elasticity** for a specific service. Price elasticity is the numerical expression of the magnitude of change in volume in response to a specific change in price, and it is represented by this formula: E = *percentage volume change ÷ Percentage price change*. If this value is less than 1 (inelastic), a fee increase will increase revenue. If it is greater than 1 (elastic), a fee increase will decrease revenue. **In both cases, raising fees will decrease volume, but depending on the level of elasticity, revenue may be either raised or lowered.**

For those who are not "number crunchers," the important principle to remember is that **if a price is elastic, revenue can be *increased* only by *lowering* the price**. Conversely, in this instance, *raising* the price *decreases* revenue. Medical fees were in the inelastic range during medicine's growth phase, but in its current mature phase, most prices are in the elastic range.

Elasticity is affected (increased or decreased) by such things as third-party payers, copayments, deductibles, noncovered services, advertising and a physician's reputation and presentation skills. When an industry becomes more competitive, as is currently happening in medicine, fees tend to become more elastic, and because of this, patient volume is sensitive even to small changes in fees.

In a fee-for-service environment, there is a different elasticity for each individual service. Therefore, if a fee (or its copayment) is changed, the effect of that change on the revenue generated by that one service needs to be monitored. In a managed care environment, every "noncovered" service will have its own level of elasticity, and each physician should estimate that level for all fees to achieve an optimum patient volume.

The most effective way to monitor the effect of fee changes on services is to set up a dynamic model using an electronic spreadsheet such as Lotus 1-2-3 or Microsoft Excel. This model should contain all the services listed on your superbill, the fee for each service and the monthly volume for each service. In addition to monitoring the effect of any fee change, this model can also be used to predict the outcome of hypothetical fee and volume scenarios by playing "What if?" While less efficient, it is also possible to monitor price and volume changes manually. It is most effective to monitor only the top 20 percent of services, those that account for 80 percent of the practice's income.

Let me illustrate the use of elasticity in the analysis of one fee change and its subsequent effect on revenue. A custom orthopaedic splint fee will be used in the example. Suppose a practitioner's fee for a custom orthopaedic splint is $300, and he dispenses 20 splints a month. The total "splint" revenue for this office is $6,000 a month. Furthermore, suppose that after raising the fee 20 percent (to $360), the volume drops 10 percent (to 18 splints a month). Monthly "splint" revenue is now $6,480. The old fee was in the inelastic range; therefore, a fee increase raised total revenue. In this example, elasticity was (10 percent ÷ 20 percent) 0.5 percent.

Now, assume that a different practitioner's "custom splint" fee is $1,000 a pair and that she also dispenses 20 splints a month (her presentation skills are better). Her "splint" revenue is $20,000 a month. She raises her fee by 20 percent to $1,200, and the volume drops 40 percent, to 12 pairs a month. Total "splint" revenue is now $14,000 a month. The old fee was in the elastic range; therefore, a fee increase decreased total revenue. Elasticity in this example is (40 percent ÷ 20 percent) 2 percent. In these two examples, the first practitioner's fee was too low and the second's may have already been at the optimum level. **This type of trial-and-error testing will enable you to come close to determining the optimum price for your services, the price with an elasticity of 1**.

Every service you provide can be monitored in this way. When you change a fee or a copayment, elasticity can be determined quickly by monitoring the monthly volume and revenue changes for **that service only**. You can achieve the ultimate goal of maximizing total revenue by optimizing price and volume for **every** service in your practice. This becomes especially important in a managed care environment.

Discounted Contracts and Profit: A Question of Margins

Do you know the lowest fee you can accept and still make a profit when faced with the decision to accept a managed care or capitated contract? More importantly, can you determine the appropriate patient volume that produces the highest profit at a discounted rate? A lack of understanding about discounted fees can lead physicians to either turn down profitable contracts or accept unprofitable ones.

A major problem in making contract decisions is that physicians receive the wrong kind of cost information from their accountants. Accounting reports provide only **total** and **average** cost data. While it is useful to know average cost, it is the wrong cost information to use when making discounted pricing decisions. For example, most physicians would conclude that they cannot make a profit contracting for additional patients at $60 an hour if their average cost is $100 an hour. This conclusion may be incorrect. The cost information necessary to make this decision accurately is marginal, not average, cost.

Marginal cost is the cost increase created by treating one more patient or one more unit of patients (a fixed volume of patients). **Marginal revenue** is the revenue received for treating one more patient or one more unit of patients. Assuming that adequate slack time for treating new patients is available, **a contract can be accepted if the marginal revenue created by treating those patients exceeds the marginal cost of treating them because, if it does, total profit will be increased**. Total profit continues to increase by adding patients up to a point where marginal cost and marginal revenue become **equal**. If patient volume increases beyond this point and marginal cost exceeds marginal revenue, total profit will decline.

While many physicians may not be familiar with the term "marginal cost," they instinctively use the concept when considering a discount. In the past, this was easier because discounting decisions usually involved a high-fee service (such as surgery or a custom product having a known lab cost). In such a case, the marginal profit (the gap between marginal revenue and marginal cost) is high and a mistake is not too costly.

Consider the following: No practitioner will discount a medical product fee to $60 (marginal revenue) when the lab fee for producing that product is $80, no matter how much slack time is available. It is not profitable to buy something and sell it for less. In this example, marginal revenue is lower than marginal cost; therefore, the discount would not be given. However, if our "usual and customary" fee was $400, we would know that a "spot" discount to a price of $300 would be profitable, and we would dispense the "product" for this fee even though we would prefer the higher fee. In making this decision, we are reasoning that the marginal revenue of $300 is higher than the marginal cost.

Discounted pricing decisions become more difficult as patient volume increases and the profit margin narrows. The marginal cost-per-patient is harder to calculate, and a mistake is more costly; however, the approach is similar to the example above. When making such a decision, you must first estimate the total cost **change** anticipated for treating the predicted increased volume of contracted patients. This cost change should include only the additional cost of supplies and any new personnel needed to manage the additional patients, phone calls and paperwork. As discussed in an earlier chapter, fixed cost should be ignored because it remains constant regardless of which decision is made.

Next, you should estimate the marginal revenue that would be produced by this contract. Again, if marginal revenue is greater than marginal cost, the contract will increase total profit. It is not crucial that you calculate an exact marginal cost, but it is important to understand the concept and use the correct framework to help in making the decision.

To gain a better understanding of these concepts, it is helpful to study the numbers side by side. This makes it easier to visualize the cost and profit dynamics with volume changes. Table One demonstrates how, as a business grows, marginal cost declines. Later, as volume and capacity related inefficiencies begin to occur, marginal cost again increases.

Notice that in this table, marginal cost almost equals marginal revenue at a patient volume of 12 "units," and total profit is the highest at this point. When volume increases beyond 12 units, total revenue increases but total profit declines. If one were to add any patients beyond 12, the price would have to be raised to make the addition of these patients profitable. This cost-and-volume relationship exists in all businesses and demonstrates why our goal should be profit rather than revenue or volume.

Table One

A	B	C	D	E*	F
Patient Volume	Marginal Revenue (Price)	Total Revenue	Marginal Cost	Total Cost	Total Profit
		A × B			C – E
0	20.1	0.0	NA	50.00	-50.0
1	20.1	20.1	15.00	65.00	-44.9
2	20.1	40.2	10.00	75.00	-34.8
3	20.1	60.3	8.00	83.00	-22.7
4	20.1	80.4	7.00	90.00	-9.6
5	20.1	100.5	6.00	96.00	4.5
6	20.1	120.6	4.00	100.00	20.6
7	20.1	140.7	4.00	104.00	36.7
8	20.1	160.8	6.00	110.00	50.8
9	20.1	180.9	10.00	120.00	60.9
10	20.1	201.0	12.00	132.00	69.0
11	20.1	221.1	16.00	148.00	73.1
12	20.1	241.2	20.00	168.00	73.2
13	20.1	261.3	22.00	190.00	71.3
14	20.1	281.4	25.00	215.00	66.4
15	20.1	301.5	30.00	245.00	56.5

* Note that the figures from column E (Total Cost) are cumulative, derived in each row by adding the marginal cost (D) to the previous Total Cost figure. You are, in effect, keeping a "running" total, adding each additional marginal cost to your total cost number.

Understanding the dynamics behind your numbers will give you insight for making pricing, volume and profit decisions. Remember, pricing and profit decisions are made "at the margin." Do not make the mistake of concluding that your marginal profit will be 40 percent if your total overhead is 60 percent. Your **total** profit margin is 40 percent, but your **marginal** profit might only be 10 percent for the new business. If this is the case, cost-cutting measures (as outlined previously) should be far more effective in increasing your total profit than an increase in patient volume. Consider that if your marginal profit for new business is 10 percent, cutting your marginal costs by 33 percent will produce the **same** amount of profit as would increasing your patient volume by 297 percent! Which goal is easier to achieve?

CHAPTER

13

Managed Care

Preparing for Managed Care

When an industry undergoes radical change, it is presented with new opportunities and new threats. Glenn Markus, a health policy consultant, has alluded to one of the most significant threats under managed care. He has stated that, "Not everyone will win; some will be excluded and lose."

In a price-competitive industry that contains a surplus of providers, losing means more than earning less money; it could mean going out of business. While this is a serious threat when considered from the perspective of the individual provider, managed care entities consider it a **desirable** and **necessary** outcome of the change process.

In an article entitled "Making Competition in Health Care Work," from the July-August issue of *Harvard Business Review*, Mr. Markus's position is supported. It is stated in the article that, "Any healthy competitive market forces the exit of substandard players, which are displaced by efficient ones. The net result is lower costs without compromising quality." Unfortunately, a managed care entity's definition of "substandard players" is certain to be different from ours.

As was mentioned earlier, whenever the "pendulum of change" swings, its momentum carries it well past the optimum point. While businesses must muddle through this suboptimal point to survive, it is important to remember that this situation exists only in the short term and that preparation must be made to compete at a less extreme position when the pendulum ultimately settles for the long term. This can be compared to shooting ducks; to hit a duck, you need to aim at a point where that duck is going to be, not where it is now.

Many doctors are mistakenly "shooting at the duck where it is now" by signing every managed care contract at any price. This strategy is apparently driven by the fear of future exclusion, and it is causing many doctors to enter into contracts at rates substantially below the level required for providing adequate patient care, often below the doctors' actual cost of providing the care.

This strategy may ultimately backfire. St. Anthony's January 1995 *Physician Capitation Report* states, "More than 90 percent of the plans surveyed indicated they use consumer complaint information in physician renewal decisions." Doctors entering into these contracts already know they will be unable to provide quality care without rationing. Over the long term, patients will not accept this type of care. Later, when reason returns to the market and patients demand better care, better access and a greater choice of physicians, these doctors may no longer be among the choices. Not only might their reputations be damaged, but this illogical strategy would have served as a distraction from initiating the difficult changes necessary to compete realistically under managed care. My advice is to let other doctors undervalue their services and enter into contracts on which they cannot possibly deliver while you focus on improving efficiency and providing quality care.

Most of us would agree that the "old" health care system could not survive without changing because it was unbalanced in favor of doctors and patients. The "new" system is equally unbalanced in favor of insurance companies and employers/payers. No system can last unless it meets the needs of patients. Ultimately, the market will stabilize. This will happen when the pendulum returns to the point at which an optimum balance is achieved among all players, including patients, providers, employers/payers and insurance companies. Survival in this environment will require lower costs and higher quality achieved through increased efficiency.

Much of what is driving doctors to "contract at any price" is the perceived threat that there is an oversupply of specialists. Since a healthy, competitive market ultimately requires that supply and demand be in equilibrium, the ratio of specialists to population is an important issue to examine in determining long-term strategy.

In an article of the July 20, 1994, issue of the *Journal of the American Medical Association,* it was stated that by the year 2000, "... there will be an overall surplus of about 165,000 patient-care physicians ... [and] the supply of specialists will outstrip the requirement by more than 60 percent." It is this type of statistic that creates alarm, and this is one reason why many specialists are currently signing "every contract at any price." Fuel was added to the fire by Keith Borglum when he stated in a recent newsletter, *California MD's Business Advisor,* that, "50 percent or more of specialists will have inadequate patient volume to maintain a practice." He recommended that doctors, "Figure out how many of your specialty will be needed in your area and do what is necessary to be one of those who survive."

There are currently 180 physicians for every population of 100,000, and some HMOs use fewer than 77 physicians for 100,000 enrollees. While these plans are able to compete with low cost, their patients have little provider choice, and their access to specialist care often requires an unacceptable wait. While such plans might be "successful" in the short term, competition will force HMO prices to stabilize over the long term. When this occurs, all HMO prices will be similar, and competition will ultimately focus on medical and service quality.

The market will ultimately select physicians capable of delivering the highest-quality care to the greatest number of patients at a competitive price. I don't believe that all physicians will be able to make the necessary changes to be successful over the long term in this managed care environment. Those who are being distracted by the short-term "noise" in the market often follow an illogical path. They are shooting at a duck that will be long gone when the pellets arrive. Meanwhile, those who are reengineering and restructuring their practices to prepare for the long-term needs of the market are aiming ahead of the duck.

Provider Selection

Before negotiating contracts or participating in managed care networks, it is important to understand what managed care organizations are looking for in a doctor. Their task is to select cost-effective, quality-conscious providers. Given an estimated 50 percent oversupply of specialists, managed care entities can be selective.

Many managed care entities solicit doctors for membership, and they will typically exclude one-third of all practitioners from membership before solicitation. While these organizations indicate that cost and utilization information have little impact on physician selection decisions, many have extensive physician claims data available to them. Claims data are run against "filters" designed to detect billing irregularities and noncompliance with contract provisions. These irregularities are compared to standards and could include such things as volume and intensity of services, frequency percentages for the ordering of tests, misuse of codes, complication rates, unbundling of surgical services, duplicate billing and excessive referrals.

Those providers who are solicited are then screened for "quality measures" such as board certification, consumer complaints and an acceptable record of hospital staff privileges. Even with this rigorous selection process, managed care entities continue to monitor the selected providers, and membership could be terminated at a later date based on patient complaints or on a doctor's lack of compliance with contract agreements. The average termination rate is approximately 5 percent.

If you wish to participate in managed care, it is essential that you begin building a long-term profile that demonstrates you are a "cost-effective, quality-conscious provider." Most managed care entities provide patients in exchange for fee discounts and compliance with strict utilization rules.

Once you are in, you will stay in based on your quality of care and compliance with the utilization requirements of the contract. **Your profit will be determined by your cost position and your efficiency in managing this larger volume of patients and paperwork**. We have previously discussed methods for improving efficiency, and the utilization of those methods will not only increase your profitability but will also provide you with a competitive advantage for negotiating contracts. The goal of this chapter is to teach you how to apply the skills you have already learned to evaluate contract profitability and volume.

Understanding Capitation: Part One

Practitioners have been forced to adapt to a variety of reimbursement methods under managed care, and the least understood of these is capitation. Providers tend to underestimate the amount of information support they will need under capitation, yet this support is the most important element necessary for success. Managed care entities have a lot of information support, but individual practitioners, who are assigned the risk, have little.

Webster's Dictionary defines capitation as, "A tax or fee of so much per head." Under managed care, it is a per capita payment that can vary by the type of service or the person covered. This payment has a fixed monthly rate, and it is based on an amount of money paid, per enrolled member, per month (PMPM). This means that if the plan's membership is 20,000 patients and the "cap rate" for a specific specialty is $0.75, the monthly payment for those services is fixed at $15,000 a month (20,000 × $0.75), regardless of member utilization.

Using the $0.75 cap rate, the physician is taking the risk that he or she can provide the contracted services (without rationing) for less than $15,000 a month. Ideally, contracts are structured to produce the highest-quality care for the lowest price, and successful contracts should reward efficient health care providers for their performance.

The Shaller Curve

Managed care's goal is to deliver the highest-quality care at the lowest possible price. Providers would like to believe that there is a linear relationship between the amount of money spent on health care and the level of quality achieved. That is, for each "unit" of money spent on health care, there should be a corresponding and equal increase in quality of care.

Up to a point, both doctors and managed care organizations agree that this is so. We intuitively know, however, that beyond some point most cause-and-effect relationships are nonlinear. After this point, a little less benefit will be returned for additional effort. This is known as the law of diminishing marginal returns. Managed care entities believe that this is the case in the relationship between money and the quality of care in a medical practice; however, they take this a step further in arguing that a point exists where each additional dollar spent actually lowers the quality of care. While doctors offer anecdotal evidence against this concept, managed care entities offer vast amounts of statistical data in support of their position.

To better understand the relationship between quality of care and the amount of money spent on care from the managed care entity's perspective, it is helpful to understand the Shaller curve (Managed Care: Graph One) on the following page. This graph was developed by Don Shaller, M.D., to visually demonstrate the relationship between cost and quality of care in medicine. The graph assumes different shapes depending on which perspective it is depicting, the provider's or the payer's. As one moves from point "A" to point "B" along the curve, providers and managed care entities agree that quality goes up in proportion to the amount of money paid out. For each unit of money spent, a unit of quality improvement is achieved.

Managed care's position is that as the amount of money spent on health care increases, there is a point (depicted on the graph as point "B") at which quality no longer improves. As each additional dollar is spent (moving horizontally along the line from "B" to "C"), quality remains constant. Regardless of additional money spent, quality remains unchanged from point "B" to point "C." Doctors disagree. They argue that quality continues to improve from "B" to "C."

Continuing on the Shaller curve beyond point "C," managed care organizations claim that quality declines as more money is spent. Presumably, this is the pattern of a system that rewards excessive and unnecessary care. Managed care entities argue that traditional fee-for-service medicine is presumed to lie somewhere along line from "C" to "D", and managed care lies along the line from "B" to "C" with capitation at point "B."

Managed Care: Graph One

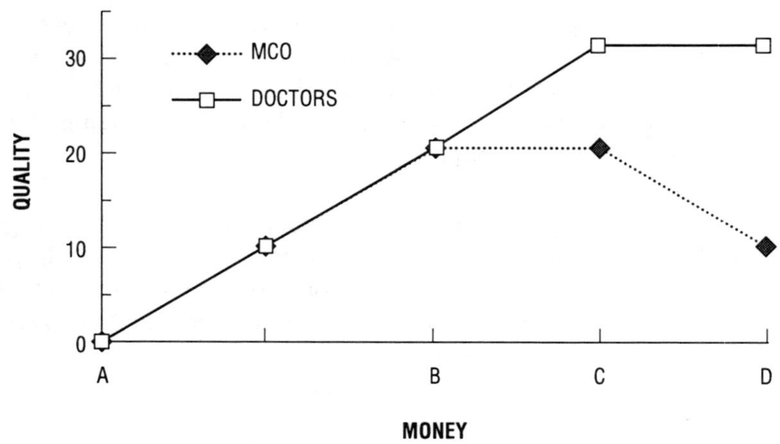

If managed care and capitation are to work over the long term, it is in the interest of both providers and managed care entities that negotiations be fair. If the capitation rate is pushed below point "B," the capitated provider will be forced to reduce quality. As long as the provider is moving along the line from "C" to "B" toward point "B," he or she is managing care and is not restricting necessary care. The managed care entity knows that this provider will ultimately reach point "B" if given enough information, education and time.

Statistics is not an exact science, and the placement of point "B" may be determined by data that are either incomplete or based on incorrect assumptions. At this time, managed care entities possess most of the available data relating to cost and quality. The only way for a group of providers to move point "B" to the right is to provide new data that prove statistically that supplying more money will produce a better quality outcome. In the absence of reliable data to prove otherwise, managed care organizations have a powerful incentive to argue that point "B" is already too far to the right. MCOs would like to move point "B" to "B1" (Managed Care: Graph Two) while physicians would prefer to move point "B" across to point "C."

Managed Care: Graph Two

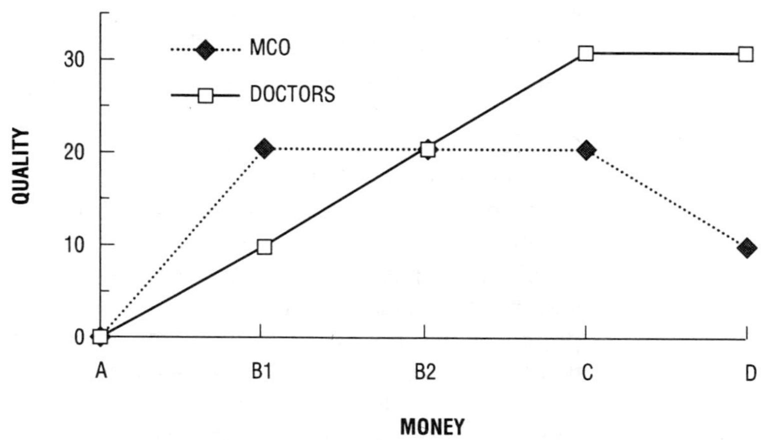

The purpose of capitation is to transfer insurance risk to the provider. Many contracts are mistakenly referred to as capitation contracts, but if there is no risk transferred to the provider, it is not a capitated contract. If a contract includes a retrospective adjustment (either up or down), which is determined at a later date, it is not a capitated contract.

The goal of managed care entities is to receive the highest-quality care at the lowest price from the provider. I do not believe that capitation will emerge as the preferred reimbursement method for the majority of specialists. One reason is that a base of at least 300,000 members is required to subcapitate all necessary specialists, smooth statistical fluctuations and stabilize risk. If membership is below 300,000, it is not possible to accurately predict the frequency at which an expensive "event" (as described below) will occur.

For example, a claim probability distribution table will demonstrate that the probability of a $200,000 "event" occurring is 1.2 per 10,000 members. This frequency is most likely to occur only if it is spread over a sufficiently large population. However, if a group is capitated with only 20,000 members, the number of members is too small for statistical fluctuations to smooth (average) out. With 20,000 members, a medical group would budget $480,000 for the predicted number of $200,000 events (1.2 × 2 × $200,000). If five such events occur, the budget will be negative by $520,000 [($200,000 × 5) - $480,000]. The chances for a $1,000,000 claim are 0.02 per 10,000. What amount should the group budget for this contingency?

For managed care groups with smaller memberships, it is likely that a budget will be developed for each specialty within the contract, and some form of global package pricing will be used. For this to work, specialists will have to develop preferred practice guidelines to control overutilization.

Even if capitation does not ultimately emerge as the preferred method of specialty reimbursement, there will be opportunities for many physicians to participate in capitated contracts. I feel that it is important to understand capitation, and if you are prepared for participation in capitation, you automatically will be prepared to compete and profit under any scenario that managed care presents.

One important element of capitation from the capitators' perspective is that sufficient control of the practitioner can be gained only by providing him or her with a large enough stream of patients to make that doctor monetarily dependent on the contract. Gaining such control enables the capitator to negotiate better rates and enforce the utilization and quality standards of the contract by threatening expulsion if the physician does not live up to the terms of the contract. Capitators feel that this is necessary because capitated providers have a financial incentive to restrict patient access, limit care, or provide substandard care. Managed care entities using statistics have determined that they need to account for at least 7.5 percent of a doctor's income if they are to have leverage (control) over that doctor. They feel that without this minimum percentage, the threat of withdrawing a contract for substandard performance is not a sufficient financial threat to the doctor.

Comparing contract "cap rates" is like comparing apples to oranges. Each contract is unique. Each one may cover a different set of services, each with its own predicted cost and utilization rate. Yet, practitioners tend to compare contracts by comparing cap rates alone.

The place to begin when calculating a profitable capitation rate is to determine the lowest possible rate at which you can provide all of the services you currently provide and still make a profit. I refer to this as the "How low can you go?" rate. If you know this number, you will automatically know that you can accept any rate higher than this.

Understanding Capitation: Part Two

There are two basic scenarios doctors will face when considering the profitability of a capitation contract. The first is when the cap rate is predetermined, and the doctor must decide if he or she can deliver the contracted services at the preestablished rate. The second is when the desired services are listed, and the doctor is asked to submit a cap rate (presumably the contract will go to the lowest bidder). We will address the scenario where the cap rate is given and the doctor must determine the contract's profitability.

As was mentioned above, contracts cannot be compared solely by their cap rates. Robert Burleigh, president of Brandywine Health Care Services in Pennsylvania, states, "Once you have seen one capitation contract, you have only seen one. No two are alike. The number of contractual variables are enormous and extremely difficult to handle." While I agree with Mr. Burleigh that no two contracts are alike and that the number of contractual variables are numerous, I feel that from a specialist's perspective, the actual number of variables relevant for estimating profitability are neither enormous nor difficult to handle.

In a competitive market, the decision to accept a contract is not based on how much profit one needs or would like but, rather, on the lowest profit margin the doctor is willing to accept (knowing that another practitioner might accept less). If a doctor is unable to determine profitability, he or she runs the risk of accepting unprofitable contracts or turning down profitable ones. The greatest risk in accepting unprofitable contracts is providing substandard care with subsequent damage to the doctor's reputation. The ultimate consequence of this might be removal of the contract. A recent survey of managed care plans indicated that 90 percent of those plans use consumer complaint information in making physician renewal decisions.

Most doctors make initial contract decisions "in the dark." Before determining a contract's profitability, it is helpful to know how MCOs calculate the capitation rates they offer. The table below illustrates how different cap rates are calculated for one specialty.

A Annual Utilization Estimate per 1,000	B Average Charge per Service	C Annual Cost per 1,000 Members	D Annual Cost per Member	E Monthly Cap Rate PMPM
		(A) × (B)	(C) ÷ 1,000	(D) ÷12
21	$32.66	$685	$0.69	$0.06
52	$88.19	$4,586	$4.59	$0.38
96	$88.75	$8,520	$8.52	$0.71

An MCO can calculate a cap rate of any amount by varying two basic assumptions, i.e., the utilization estimate and/or the average charge per service. Therefore, when given a rate, **it is important to ask the MCO what the underlying assumptions were from which the rate was derived**. The assumptions may be based on internal data, data purchased from an actuary, or a wild guess. Negotiation strategy is beyond the scope of this book, but it should be clear at this point that negotiations will be more successful when they are focused on the underlying assumptions from which the cap rate has been calculated.

Assuming that an MCO's budget is set, and the cap rate is not negotiable, the factors for determining profitability are the expected utilization per 1,000 members and the doctor's predicted increase in cost (as based on the predicted increase in patient volume created by the contract). The primary risk to the doctor is that the utilization rate might turn out to be higher than predicted. To take this risk into account, it is essential that the doctor test his or her cost-per-patient estimate over a large range of possible utilization numbers. For example, market data might demonstrate that the range of possible utilization rates for your specialty can be as low as 21, or as high as 96, per 1,000 members.

Consider the following decision: A primary care group has 20,000 patient lives under contract and is offering a capitation contract at $0.06 PMPM (per member, per month). Only nonsurgical services are included under the contract. You estimate that your average supply cost for rendering primary care services will be $2.50 per patient. The revenue for a six-cent contract will be $1,200 a month ($0.06 × 20,000 members). The next step is to test profitability against varying utilization assumptions (see table below).

A Annual Revenue	B Estimated Utilization per 1,000	C Utilization per 20,000 Members	D Variable Cost per Patient	E Total Increased Costs	F Profit
$1,200 × 12		(B) × (20)		(C) × (D)	(A) – (E)
$14,400	21	420	$2.50	$1,050	$13,350
$14,400	52	1,040	$2.50	$2,600	$11,800
$14,400	96	1,920	$2.50	$4,800	$9,600

It can be seen from the table that this contract is profitable over the entire range of utilization possibilities. The doctor might determine that he or she cannot manage the additional patient load with current office staff if utilization goes beyond 52 per 1,000. At this utilization rate, the contract would be rejected because the annual increase in cost created by hiring an additional assistant would surely be higher than the estimated profit of $11,800. The risk of this contract has now been quantified. What if variable costs-per-patient are higher? For example, what if a significant number of these patients need more involved care, requiring costlier supplies such as tape, injections, dressings, or casts? Assume that the doctor estimates the new variable cost-per-patient to be $10.00 (rather than $2.50). The table on the next page takes this new assumption into account.

A Annual Revenue	B Estimated Utilization per 1,000	C Utilization per 20,000 Members	D Variable Cost per Patient	E Total Increased Costs	F Profit
$1,200×12		(B) × (20)		(C) × (D)	(A) – (E)
$14,400	21	420	**$10.00**	$4,200	$10,200
$14,400	52	1,040	**$10.00**	$10,400	$4,000
$14,400	96	1,920	**$10.00**	$19,200	- $4,760

The above table shows that profit becomes negative beyond some point of utilization. This point can be calculated by finding the utilization rate that produces zero profit (the break-even rate). In this example, that point is at 72 per 1,000. With "B" being utilization, this can be calculated in the following way: B(20)(10) - $14,400 = $0.00; therefore, B = 72. Once this table has been established, the doctor is now in a good position to negotiate a contract. If $4,000 is the minimum profit acceptable to the doctor for servicing the contract, the doctor must then negotiate a clause which states that if utilization goes above 52 per 1,000, additional compensation will be required. If the most likely utilization rate is 52 per 1,000, the doctor may decide that cutting office costs by $4,000 (which would increase his or her profit the same amount as this contract would) would be a better choice than accepting the contract. The work required to treat an additional 1,040 patients may be more difficult than the effort necessary to cut costs by $4,000. If the contract is important to the doctor for reasons other than profit, it should be accepted only if utilization is below the break-even rate of 72 per 1,000. It is easy for a doctor to document the true cost of supplies for servicing a contract. This gives him or her leverage when negotiating a contract because he or she now has a more compelling argument for either increasing the cap rate, controlling utilization, or excluding services.

What if this same contract offered a $0.38 cap rate (producing monthly revenue of $7,600) rather than $0.06? The table on the following page depicts the change in profit using the new $0.38 cap rate and the variable cost-per-patient assumption of $10.00 used in the last example.

A Annual Revenue	B Estimated Utilization per 1,000	C Utilization per 20,000	D Variable Cost per Patient	E Total Increased Costs	F Profit
$7,600 × 12		(B) × (20)		(C) × (D)	(A) – (E)
$91,200	21	420	$10.00	$4,200	$87,000
$91,200	52	1,040	$10.00	$10,400	$80,800
$91,200	96	1,920	$10.00	$19,200	$72,000

This table demonstrates that a $0.38 contract is not overly sensitive to either utilization or supply costs. If supply costs-per-patient are less than $10.00, or utilization is "average," this is an attractive contract. If it becomes necessary to hire an additional employee, it is easy to predict the change in profit by subtracting the new employee's salary from the projected profit. At this point, it can be seen that by varying one assumption (variable) over the full range of another, any contract can be evaluated quickly for both risk and profitability.

In my office, medical supplies average 3.2 percent of the gross income. By using this percentage, the predicted supply cost for a $500,000 practice would be $16,000 ($500,000 × 0.032 = $16,000). If 3,000 patient visits are expected, the predicted average supply cost (variable cost) is $5.33 ($16,000 ÷ 3,000 = $5.33). I believe that using the medical supply cost percentage of your gross income from your annual income statement plus the salary of additional necessary employees will give a fairly accurate representation of a contract's profitability if that contract includes the same mix of services previously provided by your practice.

A "surgery only" or "procedure" contract is more complicated. Surgical utilization can be estimated by finding its percentage of the predicted overall utilization. That is, if the predicted utilization is 52 per 1,000, and experience shows that 20 percent of your patients require a procedure, then expected surgical utilization is 10.4 per 1,000, calculated as: 52 × 0.20 = 10.4. If the plan has 20,000 members, the expected number of surgeries is 208, calculated as: 10.4 × 20 = 208. Assume that the supply costs for a typical surgery are $95.00, and postoperative dressings for six visits are $15.00 (total supply cost = $110.00).

Do you accept this contract if the cap rate offered is $0.25? Monthly revenue = $5,000 a month ($0.25 × 20,000 = $5,000 monthly revenue). As before, enter the numbers into the table:

A Annual Revenue	B Estimated Utilization per 1,000	C Utilization per 20,000	D Variable Cost per Patient	E Total Increased Costs	F Profit
$5,000 × 12		(B) × (20)		(C) × (D)	(A) – (E)
$60,000	21 × **.20** = 4.20	84	**$110.00**	$9,240	$50,760
$60,000	52 × **.20** = 10.4	208	**$110.00**	$22,880	$37,120
$60,000	96 × **.20** = 19.2	384	**$110.00**	$42,880	$17,120

What if your past experience is that surgical utilization is 30 percent rather than 20 percent? Simply test this risk by recalculating profit, changing 20 percent (when estimating utilization per 1,000) to 30 percent. If you estimate that supply costs will be higher, test that new number. Continue testing risk by changing any variable that you feel uncomfortable with until you have quantified the extent of the risk. If you determine that the risk is unacceptable, use this same exercise to determine the minimum cap rate that would be acceptable to you. If you are unable to negotiate an increase in the cap rate or to control utilization of surgical services, the contract should be turned down.

One cost not included in the above surgical table is opportunity cost. Unlike a primary care contract, opportunity costs are significant when considering a surgical contract. When performing a surgical procedure, you are unavailable to provide other services at that same time. You are giving up the "opportunity" to treat other patients, and this lost opportunity is lost income that should be quantified. Obviously, if your time is currently occupied treating patients only 20 hours a week, then there is no lost opportunity; however, if your schedule is busy, a surgical contract may reduce other income or restrict other opportunities. Using the contract above, if you performed 208 surgeries and averaged two hours away from the office per surgery (travel and operating time), this would use a total of 416 hours. If postoperative visits averaged six per patient and required 15 minutes each, add another 312 hours (728 total hours). If you work 40 hours a week, 728 hours (or 18 weeks) represents one-third of your available yearly time!

A final scenario to consider is a situation where the managed care entity requests a "blind bid." They reveal to the provider only the number of patient lives under contract and the specialty services desired, and ask the provider to bid a cap rate (presumably the contract will go to the lowest bidder). In this situation, the place to begin is to determine the break-even cap rate at different levels of expected utilization. Assume that this contract has 20,000 members and that only nonsurgical services are required. In this example, assume utilization to be 52 per 1,000 and variable cost to be $4.62 per patient.

For this example (Where R = revenue and C = Costs):

$$R = \textit{cap rate} \times 20{,}000 \times 12$$
$$C = \$4.62 \times 52 \times 20.$$

The break-even cap rate will be the cap rate at which:

$$R - C = 0$$
$$\therefore (\textit{cap rate} \times 20{,}000 \times 12) - (\$4.62 \times 52 \times 20) = 0$$
$$\textit{Cap rate} = (\$4.62 \times 52 \times 20) \div (20{,}000 \times 12) = 0$$
$$\therefore \textit{Break-even cap rate} = \$0.02 \textit{ PMPM}$$

If the contract is for surgery only, repeat this exercise by inserting the variable cost and utilization rate (52 per 1,000) from the previous example.

$$\textit{Revenue} = \textit{cap rate} \times 20{,}000 \times 12.$$
$$\textit{Cost} = \$110 \times 10.4 \times 20$$

The break-even surgery cap rate will be the cap rate at which:

$$R - C = 0$$
$$\therefore (\textit{Cap rate} \times 20{,}000 \times 12) - (\$110 \times 10.4 \times 20) = 0$$
$$\textit{Cap rate} = (\$110 \times 10.4 \times 20) \div (20{,}000 \times 12) = \$0.10$$
$$\therefore \textit{Break-even surgery cap rate} = \$0.10 \textit{ PMPM}$$

The surgical break-even cap rate is $0.10, but this ignores opportunity costs. It is up to each individual doctor to determine the level of profit he or she is willing to accept in order to "win" a contract. By inserting the desired profit number into tables, as discussed above, a doctor can easily work back and determine the cap rate that will produce the desired profit.

It is important to recognize that in the current competitive marketplace, there are few opportunities for specialists to negotiate fees. Fees are generally set in advance by managed care organizations and are determined by the marketplace. When Blue Cross reduced fees paid to specialists for the fourth straight year, David Chernof, Blue Cross medical director, replied, "The **fee adjustments reflect what consumers**, from individuals to large corporations, **are willing to pay for health care**." This is similar to other services or products that are in oversupply; if the supplier cannot meet the market price, he or she is "out of the market."

As a final consideration before accepting any contract, one should always compare the contract's expected profit to the equivalent savings that could be produced by reducing costs. For example, I previously presented an example of a contract with a $0.06 cap rate that produced $9,600 profit. If this contract was "won" by the doctor, it would require that he or she manage an additional 1,920 patient visits a year. For a $500,000 practice, this $9,600 profit would be equivalent to the savings produced by a modest 1.92 percent cost-reduction. This might be the better path to pursue. Remember, **cost-reduction through efficiency improvement is the key to competing profitably under managed care**. An efficient practitioner has a reduced need for accepting low-margin contracts, and if he or she does accept such contracts, they will result in more profit.

Where Are Capitation Rates Headed?

In 1994, the Advisory Board Company reported the results of a survey of specialty capitation rates representing 62 percent of the commercial HMO population. The table below gives the results of that survey for 12 specialties.

SPECIALTY	AVERAGE PMPM
Anesthesiology	$1.771
Cardiology	$0.636
Cardiology (invasive)	$0.361
General Surgery	$1.101
Neurology	$0.264
OB/GYN	$2.305
Oncology	$0.274
Ophthalmology	$0.695
Orthopaedics	$1.159
Psychiatry/Psychology	$1.671
Radiology	$1.910
Urology	$0.497

A recent survey representing 183 capitated contracts from 37 managed care plans estimated the average cap rate for one specialty to be $0.218 PMPM. The rates in this survey ranged from a low of $0.04 to a high of $0.68 PMPM. For the $0.218 rate to be profitable, there are two requirements: 1) the contract must represent only a small percentage of a practice's total volume; and 2) the doctor must be able to spread the increased patient volume across existing fixed costs. While this rate can be profitable when applied to a small percentage of a practice's patient volume, it is not profitable if applied to the majority of the practice.

If capitation should grow to become the reimbursement method for the majority of a practice's patient volume, a doctor might ask, "What should my average cap rate be?" To answer this question, let's first look at what would happen if the rate from the above example remained unchanged. If the $0.218 average cap rate is applied using the current ratio of this specialty to population (one per 20,000), this would produce an annual gross income for each physician of $52,320, calculated as: $0.218 × 20,000 × 12. This is one-fourth of the $208,000 median gross income reported for this specialty in 1994.

One might surmise from the above data that three-fourths of this specialty would not survive the 21-cent cap rate. The remaining one-fourth would need to be able to treat four times its previous volume of patients. Even if quality is ignored, the quadrupling of patient volume to produce the same $208,000 gross income would increase overhead costs substantially and eliminate most, if not all, of the profit. Under this scenario, even the contract "winners" are "losers."

By using the 1994 gross income figure, one can calculate that $208,000 represents an inferred cap rate of 87 cents PMPM, calculated as: 20,000 × $0.87 × 12 = $208,800, four times the current average rate of $0.218. While 21 cents is too low to become the "final" rate, a return to the 87-cent rate is equally unlikely. I believe that over the long term, the health care industry will follow the same pattern as have all other industries that have undergone a highly competitive period; prices for health care coverage will stabilize at some level, and competition will again focus on quality. I predict that at that point, cap rates for the above example will be around 61 cents, 30 percent lower than their previous high of 87 cents. While this is better than 21 cents, only efficient practices will thrive in this environment. I believe that this **30 percent cost-reduction target applies to all practitioners** who wish to survive the long-term financial impact of managed care.

A cost-reduction of this magnitude requires an aggressive combination of efficiency techniques and possible joint ventures with other practitioners. Effective joint ventures may be partial (business office only) or complete practice mergers. If done properly, overhead can be cut dramatically and the joint venture is better positioned to compete for managed care contracts.

Regardless of what form managed care ultimately assumes, the foundation of every practitioner's long-range strategic plan should be efficiency improvement. Efficiency is important even if practices merge, because combining two or more inefficient practices will produce one large inefficient practice with no significant cost savings. If it turns out that capitation rates end up settling at a higher figure than I have predicted here (and I hope they do) or if managed care is outlawed by Congress, efforts directed at change will not be in vain because efficient practices will still achieve higher quality, be able to treat more patients with less waste and be rewarded with higher profit.

CHAPTER

14

Mergers and Acquisitions

Mergers and Acquisitions: Optimizing Office Space

When other industries are confronted with price competition similar to what medicine currently faces, they utilize various competitive strategies for survival. Some companies become "leaner and meaner" by improving operational efficiency and downsizing their operations, while others either merge with other companies or sell out to larger organizations.

We have discussed methods for improving operational efficiency with the goal of reducing total overhead expenses. If fees or patient volume continue to decline, the possibility of a merger or acquisition will make sense for some practitioners. While there are many examples of practitioners who have acquired practices and run multiple offices, there are few examples of successful mergers; however, a merger of medical practices has more opportunities for lowering overhead than does an acquisition.

Successful, long-term partnerships in medicine are difficult. There are many reasons for this, but the most common are differences in individual productivity, differences in treatment and practice philosophies, or lack of a personality "fit." I overheard one of my favorite quotes related to the productivity problem when a doctor on a hospital elevator asked, "Why is it that every doctor is a workaholic except for my partner?"

There appears to be a growing national consensus that the traditional solo practitioner will have difficulty surviving under managed care unless he or she is able to affiliate with a larger group practice. Mergers are generally driven by a belief that overhead can be reduced by combining several practices into one facility, thereby eliminating redundant activities and spreading patient volume over the same, or lower, fixed costs. While this goal is attainable when both practices are efficient, **combining two or more inefficient practices could create one large inefficient practice incapable of achieving the expected cost savings**.

Many busy practices have experienced dramatic reductions in revenues with no corresponding reduction in costs. In these cases, practice overhead that was once 50 to 60 percent of revenues may go above 80 percent. Even with such severe financial hardship, these practices often continue to treat large volumes of patients. If several practices in close proximity are experiencing this problem, practice mergers should be considered.

While there are many important considerations to remember when contemplating a merger, the most important is to streamline (reengineer) and merge business systems before merging the practices. Once this is accomplished, a compensation system needs to be developed that rewards both productivity and cost-reductions. One way to accomplish this is to establish the same fixed overhead for each doctor (e.g., 60 percent of revenues collected) and place it in a pooled overhead account. All expenses are paid out of this account, and any funds remaining in this account are distributed equally at a later time. This method recognizes that each doctor will have a different size practice and a different level of productivity. It also recognizes that the higher the revenue an individual doctor generates, the greater his or her impact will be on costs. The most important features of this strategy are that all the doctors have an equal incentive to keep costs under control, unequal productivity is accounted for and the potential for negative consequences that could result from internal competition among the doctors for new patients and higher paying procedures is reduced.

One alternative to the "traditional" merger is a hybrid that allows each doctor to retain his or her autonomy. The specific type of merger that I feel can accomplish this and still help address the cost problems associated with the managed care market is the merger of medical business offices. This option addresses cost issues without adding many of the problems associated with a total practice merger. Our most formidable competition is the HMO staff model that consists of many individual practitioners working in the same building with one business office. Compare this with a building, such as yours or mine, where many doctors practice, each with an individual business office. Which method do you think is more cost-effective?

The following trends in private practice should be reason for alarm: 1) the business office space in most offices constitutes a larger percentage of the total office space than it did in the past; and 2) there has been a shift in the distribution of staff from the back to the front of the office to address the increasing volume and complexity of paperwork. These trends mean that **an increasing amount of money is being spent for office space and office staff to perform nonmedically-productive and nonbillable services. This problem will worsen as patient volumes increase and fees decline further.**

Rent and staff salaries are the two largest expenses in private practice. A merger of business offices presents the opportunity to reduce office and staff size if volume is decreasing, or to redistribute staff and office space toward more productive patient care activities if patient volume is increasing. Each practice may have special needs (such as a person who follows up on payment denials) that do not require a full-time person. Several merged offices could afford to employ such a person full-time by sharing the salary expense.

I feel that merging business offices is a better alternative than outsourcing insurance billing. Most billing services charge a high percentage based on the money collected, and their collection percentage tends to be lower than in-office billing. Doctors are often reluctant to give up control of the billing function, and a merger can create a scenario where the distraction of the billing activities is out of the office, the doctor does not give up control and the cost is much lower. The more business offices that merge, the lower the cost, and there is no specific limit to the number of offices that can be merged.

To gain the maximum benefit and efficiency from a merger, it is necessary to use the efficiency concepts that we have discussed. Rather than marking a superbill, the doctor should enter the diagnosis and treatment charges directly into an office computer terminal. At the end of the day, this information would be transferred to a disk or electronically transmitted to the central billing office. The billing information in the office computer would always be current. It would be accessible to discuss a bill with a patient and to collect the balance due while the patient was in the office. This is the same level of control as having individual, in-office billing.

In addition to insurance billing, there may be other business office functions that could be more cost-effective if shared. Competitive strategies in the future will need to include "rethinking" traditional business practices that have been successful in the past but may not fit today's economic models. Creative merging of business office functions presents one alternative strategy for lowering costs without lowering quality. Forming a "group practice without walls" is an important strategy that combines the cost savings from merging business operations with the contracting advantages of a large group practice. It requires giving up autonomy, but the potential gain may be worth the effort. Forming a group practice without walls is beyond the scope of this book, but understanding and implementing the efficiency concepts discussed in the book are essential for its success.

CHAPTER

15

The Accounts Payable Process and Accounting

Computerized Check Writing for the Accounts Payable Process

Under managed care, it is becoming important to have detailed financial data regarding costs. As data accumulate in paper form, it becomes increasingly difficult to find and retrieve relevant financial data when the information is needed. Computerized check writing is essential for this task, and if done correctly, it can also substantially reduce accounting costs.

I recall paying bills with a manual system that required a tedious process of disbursing each payment to its appropriate account, totaling 30 accounts as each page was completed and reconciling the checking account with the monthly bank statement. The system provided no vendor history or other useful data necessary for analyzing trends or making comparisons.

At the end of each month, I would "dump" all the information at my accountant's office, and he would check my work, make journal entries and produce financial statements. While the financial statements were interesting to review, they were old news by the time I received them. I would also receive a bill from my accountant for the work performed.

After I converted to a computerized check-writing system, I realized how fast I could spend money! I no longer had to total expense accounts, and reconciling the checking account was easier. I felt well organized the first time that I was able to hand my accountant a neatly typed check register and legible reports, but in spite of the more detailed information that I gave him, my accounting expenses went up. Part of his explanation was that he had to enter my data into his computer, make journal entries, produce a general ledger and check my work.

My accounting fees continued to escalate and I began to question the value of my accountant's service. The reports I received from my computer were more timely than his, and there appeared to be much duplication of effort. CPAs are vital to the operation of public companies, which need to assure stockholders that their financial data are true and accurate; however, medical practices don't have stockholders. With the exception of income and payroll taxes, financial matters of medical practices are of concern only to the doctors who run those practices.

When my accounting fees reached an unacceptable level, I found a new CPA. I asked this CPA which software she used. Her software was more sophisticated than mine, but I determined that it could be learned easily. Upon converting to the new system, I immediately saved money because I was able to give her a disk containing my accounting information, and this could be imported directly into her system. I was also able to control cash-flow better because invoices were entered into the computer as they arrived. This made it possible for me to keep up-to-date information on accounts payable, and checks were automatically printed in order of due dates.

Over time, I realized that this system performed many of the functions I was paying my accountant to complete, including producing a detailed, double-entry journal and all financial statements. By simply using my computer to "pay bills," all standard accounting procedures and reports were completed automatically, and I could generate any report I needed. I have now personally taken over all accounting duties for my office except for payroll and filing income taxes. I found it cheaper and easier to transfer payroll to a service, and my CPA still does my tax returns better and faster than I can.

Most doctors use computerized check-writing systems, but many are using systems designed for home use rather than business use. Some doctors are intimidated by the "accounting jargon" used in an accounting software manual and necessary for setting up expense accounts; however, once a system is established, little accounting knowledge is needed. If you are involved in other businesses, this same software can accommodate all of them. This is important because many hobbies become businesses, and accounting fees can eat up much of the profit.

I prefer to pay my office bills outside the office; however, if bills are paid in the office, it is more difficult for funds to be embezzled when accounting software is used. A detailed paper trail always exists and entries cannot be erased or changed. If a mistake is made, standard accounting procedures require reversing the journal entry by crediting and debiting the appropriate accounts. This affects four separate expense accounts, making it difficult to alter any individual account. Accounting software also makes the unauthorized use of checks difficult by requiring an accurate accounting of all voided and missing checks.

While different practitioners may prefer the unique features of one check-writing program over another, all programs are capable of improving the accounts payable process; however, in today's price-competitive medical environment, I believe that simply improving a process is not enough. We have seen how other office processes can be improved and made less costly, and the accounts payable process is no exception. The main barrier for most physicians is that they have developed the habit of using the services of a CPA for all routine accounting matters. If you are already using a computer check-writing program, the next step is to determine which of your accounting needs you have an accountant fulfill. Then, as in my example of payroll, determine whether a CPA is the most cost-effective provider for that service. I believe that by rethinking your accounts payable process, you can decrease your accounting costs by at least 85 percent.

CHAPTER

16

Inventory Management

Cash Flow and the ABC Inventory Method

In every business, there are times when money runs out before the bills are paid. This is referred to as a cash-flow problem, and even highly profitable medical practices experience such problems. These times are usually temporary and are handled by simply delaying payment on selected bills until enough money comes in to cover them. Under managed care, cash-flow problems may occur more frequently, and we need to direct more attention toward reducing their frequency and severity.

While it is obvious that some causes of cash-flow problems are not under our direct control, we should seek to control those that are. The money that we have available to pay bills is part of our working capital. While we tend to think of working capital as the cash we have in the bank, it also includes other current assets such as inventory. Unlike cash, inventory is not usable for paying bills or purchasing equipment. If cash flow is a frequent problem, one strategy a practitioner can use to “free up” some cash is to reduce the amount of working capital that is tied up in the form of excess inventory.

Inventory management and cash-flow management are interrelated. Unfortunately, doctors typically spend more time tracking and categorizing inventory than managing it. They tend to accumulate a safety stock of inventory to protect against the danger of running out of supplies. Although a practice must maintain sufficient quantities of inventory to meet the demands of its operations, it is desirable to keep the amount of cash invested in inventory to a minimum because inventories in excess of business needs tie up funds unnecessarily. To offset declines in revenue created by managed care, some doctors are beginning to increase medical supply inventory to sell to patients. While this may eventually increase revenue, this larger inventory needs to be managed carefully to prevent accompanying cash-flow and storage problems.

For most companies, the expenses associated with financing and maintaining inventories are a substantial part of the cost of doing business. Accordingly, it makes sense for large companies to spend a significant amount of time managing inventory. It is important to track each item to determine inventory holding costs, the cost of placing orders and the frequency of reordering. While there are sophisticated computer programs and models that assist large companies in tracking and managing inventories, they can be too unnecessarily complicated and time consuming to benefit a typical medical practice.

In a medical office, the primary economic impacts created by excess inventory are the reduction of cash flow and the increased need for storage space. Most practices have noncomputerized processes in place that are adequate for tracking inventory, determining when to order items and knowing how much of each item to order. There are, however, hundreds of items in our inventories, and they do not affect cash flow and storage space equally. As was discussed earlier, given limited time and resources, we should develop a strategy that focuses on those few items that have the greatest cost impact.

The simplest method for managing inventory, and one that provides the biggest "bang for the buck," is the A-B-C method of stratifying inventory by total annual expenditure. You must first identify the "A" items in your inventory. These are the 10 percent to 20 percent of the items in the inventory that account for 70 to 80 percent of your inventory costs. Next, identify the "C" items. These are the 70 to 80 percent of the items that account for only 5 to 10 percent of costs. The "B" items are those remaining. The strategy is to focus on the "A" items first, followed by the "B's." Order smaller quantities of these items more often, and negotiate prices and delivery schedules more aggressively.

Computerized spreadsheets are the ideal type of software for stratifying inventory in order of cost. If each inventory item and the annual expense for that item is entered onto a computer spreadsheet, your inventory list can be instantly sorted in descending order by total annual cost. The cost of each item on the list can then be compared to the cost of total inventory and categorized as an "A," "B," or "C" item.

Time and effort spent on identifying the "A" items in your inventory is productive because the information gained will help free up cash and storage space. It is also valuable to comparison-shop or negotiate a better price for these items or, if price is firm, to negotiate advantageous services such as shorter lead times for ordering or lower shipping costs. Another possibility is to form a group of doctors (possibly a local society) that is able to offer a higher volume of business to a vendor in exchange for lower prices and/or an advantageous delivery schedule.

Typical inventory categories in a medical office include business office supplies and medical supplies. These constitute 5 percent of total costs in my office; however, I have consulted for offices where medical supplies alone accounted for almost 10 percent of total office costs. Expensive or bulky customized products should be included as an inventory "A" item because they have high lab fees and shipping costs, and delayed deliveries or prolonged storage of a product waiting to be dispensed ties up a great deal of working capital and creates storage problems.

With such a large number of inventory items, the goal is to "keep it simple." Don't waste valuable time shopping for better prices, negotiating discounts or monitoring the majority of your inventory (the "C" items). You can keep the software simple, too, with an easy-to-use, computerized spreadsheet. While inventory management will not solve all of your cash-flow problems, it can be structured to help you avoid some of them.

Epilogue

The concepts and tools taught in this book remain constant in an environment of change. Given a future in which the only constant will be change, doctors will be faced with making decisions under conditions of uncertainty. Most of the decisions you will be facing will not have a textbook solution, but you will be able to use these new tools to develop the best solutions possible using the data available. Every decision involves weighing potential risks and rewards, and possessing the skills to contain risk will give you the confidence to face each new decision as it arises.

You cannot eliminate all risk from a decision, but it can be contained at an acceptable level. Not every decision will turn out to be the best one, but if you understand and use the concepts taught in this book, you will make better decisions consistently. The effects of making better decisions accumulate over the long term and will result in rewards that outweigh risks by an ever-increasing margin. You will find that by rereading this book, you will gain an even better understanding of the concepts and will have added confidence with which to face an uncertain future.

Many of the efficiency "solutions" suggested in this book involve the application of computer networks. I find it interesting that *Business Week* magazine, June 26, 1995, devoted its first annual report on information technology to the "Networked Corporation." This report concluded that a network of computers is fast becoming a necessity for competing in business but that not all companies are successfully applying computer networks to achieve lower costs and improved customer service. The *Business Week* report cautions, "Networks do not an efficient workplace make." In other words, companies are discovering that simply networking computers will not automatically create efficiency benefits. After reading this book, I believe that you could advise many of these companies as to why they have not achieved greater efficiency using their networks.

It was gratifying for me to review a report from the Conference Board that came out just after I finished this book. The report was entitled, "Purchasing Value in Health Care" and was written for the largest purchasers of health care in the United States, big business. According to the Conference Board's CEO, Jack V. Wirts, this report was made in an attempt to find practical solutions for companies and providers who want to control costs while maintaining quality. The report recommended purchasing "value" and defined value as the following: "A combination of outstanding clinical quality, outstanding service quality and cost-effectiveness. Health care systems must focus on the improvement of all three." I believe that all three can be accomplished through efficiency improvement and, as this becomes the goal for all health care purchasers, doctors who understand the contents of this book will be well-positioned to thrive under managed care.

After gaining the necessary knowledge and skills for improving efficiency, the greatest barrier to implementing an efficiency program for a large company often lies in its company culture. While change is always difficult, many companies have management styles in place that create significant barriers for using networks effectively. What is true for large companies can also be true for small businesses such as medical practices. The latest buzzword in business today is *Open-Book Management*, which is a way of running a company that gets everyone focused on helping the business make money. Management techniques such as TQM and reengineering give employees tools but only teach *how*. Open-Book Management works because it teaches employees *why*. Employees need to know both *how* and *why* if they are to have the independent motivation and skills needed to help make change happen. It should be obvious from the name that Open-Book Management implies trust and free access to information. These conditions are essential if the greatest gains are to be achieved using networks.

Two years ago, I had a conversation with a physical therapist who complained about his high overhead. He had six offices, but he had achieved no cost savings using a centralized billing operation. I suggested that he could cut costs significantly by entering data directly into the computer from each office location rather than on paper superbills. This one change would not only have eliminated four data entry people, it would have eliminated transportation and storage of superbills, thus cutting a week's delay in initiating his billing cycle. He explained that this would not work in his operation because the employees working at each office would see how much he charged! Obviously, this is not Open-Book Management. It leaves few opportunities for developing innovative network solutions to his high-cost problems. It also explains why so many of my patients had complained to me about difficulties with bills they had received from this therapist's central billing office.

Computer networks add less value when they are applied in a "closed-book" environment. Changing an office culture can be difficult, but it is as important as changing technology. To achieve optimum benefits from using computer networks, employees need to be cross-trained, empowered and trusted. Without cross-training, computer applications cannot be applied from different locations simultaneously. Without empowerment, employees cannot take the initiative to apply their skills at the moment they are needed or to assist with improving processes. Without trust, employees become the "enemy," and they cannot help in achieving office goals.

Appendixes One and *Two* contain two articles written by my brother, Kenneth Hultman, on the topic of change as it relates to employee involvement. They were written for larger organizations, but I believe they apply equally well to any business contemplating change. Ken is certified as a training consultant specializing in individual and team performance and organizational change.

APPENDIX

1

"Removing Barriers to Organizational Change"

By Kenneth E. Hultman, Ed.D.

To remain competitive, change is critical, and resistance to change can be crippling. Therefore, the ability to diagnose and deal with resistance has emerged as an essential skill for supervisors, managers and others responsible for leading people through change. This article will help you increase your expertise in this area by examining the symptoms and causes of resistance, outlining an approach for diagnosing resistance and offering solutions for lowering resistance.

Symptoms and Causes of Resistance

Symptoms are the specific behaviors people use to resist change, and fall into two categories—**ACTIVE** and **PASSIVE** resistance. Some examples of behaviors in each category are as follows:

ACTIVE RESISTANCE		
Being critical	*Blaming/accusing*	*Blocking*
Fault-finding	*Sabotaging*	*Undermining*
Ridiculing	*Intimidating*	*Starting rumors*
Appealing to fear	*Manipulating*	*Arguing*
Using facts selectively		*Distorting facts*

PASSIVE RESISTANCE
Agreeing verbally but not following through.
Failing to implement change.
Procrastinating/dragging feet.
Feigning ignorance
Withholding information, suggestions, help or support.
Standing by and allowing the change to fail.

These behaviors tell us that people are resisting change, but they don't tell us **why**. To diagnose the causes, we must understand a person's state of mind. The most important factors making up one's state of mind are his or her facts, beliefs, feelings and values. These factors can be defined as follows:

FACTS are objective realities that can be proven with evidence such as *"I've worked here 15 years."*

BELIEFS are subjective assumptions, conclusions, and predictions.

> **Assumption:** *"I'm valuable to the organization because I've been here a long time."*
>
> **Conclusion:** *"I don't need to learn new skills."*
>
> **Prediction:** *"My job will be safe."*

FEELINGS represent our emotions *("I get angry when I'm told I have to change.")*

VALUES are beliefs about what's important. Values represent the criteria we use to evaluate alternatives and our priorities *"I place a lot of emphasis on loyalty."*

If we take people's state of mind into consideration, the six most common causes of resistance to change are as follows:

1. **They believe their needs are being met already.** In other words, they have no incentive or motivation to change because they're content with the way things are now. As long as this is true, change will only be viewed as negative.

2. **They believe the change will make it harder for them to meet their needs.** As such, they see the change as a threat, instead of something that could be helpful. In situations like these, facts tend to be less significant than the beliefs (assumptions, conclusions and predictions) stemming from them. It's normal for people to be concerned about how they're going to be affected by change, but unviable, pessimistic beliefs about bad things happening are damaging because they are often based on inaccurate, incomplete, or mistaken information. These beliefs lead to fear and values that emphasize protecting oneself against the perceived threat.

3. **They believe the risks outweigh the benefits.** Resistance is neither inherently good nor bad. It's adaptive and healthy for people to resist harmful change. Our focus, however, is on situations where people believe the change is harmful when this isn't actually true. As long as they believe the risks outweigh the benefits, they'll be afraid of the change and try to defend themselves against it.

4. **They believe change is unnecessary to avoid or escape a harmful situation.** A lot of the changes being introduced in U.S. organizations now are in response to increased competition from other countries. Leaders maintain these changes are necessary to survive, but a lot of employees simply don't believe this. Instead they believe the changes are just another way to get more work out of them. These employees are in denial; it's important for them to face realities, or be left behind.

5. **They believe the change process was handled improperly.** People are not only capable of resisting the change itself, but also the methods used to bring the change about. This can happen if they had no input into the decision, they don't like how the change was introduced, the change was a surprise, the timing of the change was bad, or they feel manipulated and deceived by management. People react to things like this with anger because the methods used go against their values. We live in an age when employees expect to have their views considered and to be treated with respect. Even the most constructive change can backfire if we don't remember this.

6. **They believe the change will fail.** People can resist change because they don't have confidence it will work or they don't believe the resources are available to implement the change successfully. The anxiety stemming from these concerns will make it more difficult for people to support the change effort.

Diagnosing Resistance

Since we can't literally *see* a person's state of mind, it must be inferred from what he or she says and does. Therefore, when observing what someone does, ask yourself, *"What fact, belief, feeling, or value is being reflected by what this person is doing?"* Similarly, when listening to someone, ask yourself, *"What fact, belief, feeling or value is being conveyed by what this person is saying?"*

Although it's possible for resistance to stem from a single fact, belief, feeling or value, this is the exception. In addition, there is the danger of identifying a symptom rather than the cause of resistance. Facts, beliefs, feelings and values are usually linked together in sequences or patterns. The most effective way to find missing pieces in a pattern is to ask nonthreatening questions relevant to the specific situation. Some examples are:

FACTS

- What information are you basing that on?
- How do you know that's true?
- What evidence do you have?
- How did you arrive at that conclusion?
- What facts do you have to back that up?

BELIEFS

- What's your opinion of this change?
- Do you think this change will work? Why not?
- What problems do you see with this change?
- Why else don't you think we should make this change?
- What do you think is going to happen?

FEELINGS

- How does that make you feel?
- What are your concerns about this?
- I can see you're upset, can we talk about it?
- You sound angry, can we discuss the situation?
- It looks like something's bothering you. Do you want to tell me about it?

VALUES

- What's important to you about how this is handled?
- What outcomes do you want to see from this change?
- What's the bottom line for you?
- How would you prefer that we deal with this?
- What criteria do you think we should use to evaluate alternatives?
- What are your priorities?

Effectively Dealing with Resistance

Generally speaking, overcoming resistance is a process of:

(1) **Verifying** facts,

(2) **Challenging** beliefs,

(3) **Acknowledging** feelings, and

(4) **Relating** the change to people's values.

There is, however, no formula for instant success. As we've seen, resistance has a variety of possible causes, and individuals resist change for different reasons. Therefore, it's important to tailor your approach to each situation. Earlier, six reasons were discussed why people are unreceptive to change. Some suggestions for dealing with each reason are as follows:

1. **They believe their needs are being met already.**
    - Explain why the change is necessary.
    - Indicate how the change will allow them to meet their needs better.
    - Determine if they're setting their sights too low.
    - Discover if they're holding back due to fear of losing something.

2. **They believe the change will make it harder for them to meet their needs.**
   - Discover if their facts are accurate and complete.
   - Determine if their beliefs are based on accurate information.
   - Provide additional information to correct mistaken or inaccurate beliefs.
   - Offer more viable interpretations of the facts.
   - Ask them what positive results they think can come out of the change.
   - Suggest ways you could make the change easier for them.
   - Ask how you can help them implement the change.
   - Ask for suggestions on how to make the change work better.
   - Ask for alternatives to the change that might be more effective.
   - Follow through on agreements reached to improve the situation.

3. **They believe the risks outweigh the benefits.**
   - Ask them to discuss the risks.
   - Determine if the risks are based on accurate information.
   - Provide additional information to correct inaccurate or mistaken beliefs.
   - Offer more viable interpretations of the facts.
   - Listen and respond to their issues and concerns.
   - Point out how the benefits of the change relate to their values.

4. **They believe change is unnecessary to avoid or escape a harmful situation.**
   - Provide facts about the current condition of the organization and the competition.
   - Explain how the change will help the organization survive and grow.
   - Listen and respond to their issues and concerns.
   - Ask for their support in making the change work.

5. **They believe the change process was handled improperly.**
   - Ask for and listen to their concerns.
   - Apologize for mistakes, or the issue will never go away.
   - Provide additional information (not excuses) as needed.
   - Ask for suggestions to avoid similar situations in the future.
   - Be honest about suggestions you can and cannot accept, and indicate why. People appreciate a straight answer.
   - Follow through on agreements reached to improve the situation. If people believe they've been given the brush-off, it will make things much worse.

6. **They believe the change will fail.**
    - Ask for and listen to their concerns.
    - Discover if their facts are accurate and complete.
    - Determine if their beliefs are based on accurate information.
    - Provide additional information to correct mistaken or inaccurate beliefs.
    - Offer more viable interpretations of the facts.
    - Ask for suggestions to help make the change successful.
    - Ask for alternatives to the change that might be more effective.
    - Ask how you can help them implement the change.
    - Follow through on agreements reached to improve the situation.
    - Ask for their support in making the change work.

Implementing these suggestions effectively will allow you to remove barriers to change, providing a clear path toward organizational success.

APPENDIX

2

Trust: A Key to Team Success

By Kenneth E. Hultman, Ed.D.

When I work as a facilitator with teams experiencing interpersonal conflict, the members almost always tell me privately that they don't trust each other. Trust is a key factor contributing to team productivity, quality, morale and organizational growth; mistrust, on the other hand, saps the team of valuable time and energy, contributing to organizational suicide. The problem with mistrust is that it operates insidiously below the surface and, instead of dealing with it directly, people often build their work around it. With increasing competition, however, the assumption that mistrust can be tolerated is no longer viable. A basis for trust must be established if a team is to have any hope of developing its full potential. This article will shed some light on this important topic by: (1) discussing the dynamics of trust and mistrust; (2) describing actions leading to mistrust; and (3) offering some suggestions for enhancing team trust.

The Dynamics of Trust

Trust can be defined as believing another person has your best interests at heart, whereas mistrust is believing that the other person doesn't have your best interests at heart. Mistrust is a feeling that the other person is trying to control or manipulate you to their end, rather than sharing control to accomplish some joint end. Trust is a dynamic variable that fluctuates up or down, depending on how we interpret another person's behavior. Thus, it's possible to trust someone to a greater extent one minute and less the next. We make adjustments like this on a conscious or subconscious basis all the time as we interact with other people.

Trust is an **output** that depends on certain **inputs**. In deciding whether or not to trust someone (the output), we evaluate their behavior according to its consistency and sincerity (the inputs). Consistency has to do with whether or not the other person is ethical, reliable and dependable. The question we ask ourselves here is, *"Can I count on this person to do the right thing?"* Sincerity has to do with whether or not the other person is genuine and non-manipulative. The question we ask ourselves here is, *"Can I count on this person to be really concerned about me?"* Consistency focuses on the predictability of the other person's observable behavior. Sincerity focuses on the other person's motives, which can't be directly observed but must be inferred from their verbal and non-verbal behavior. Trust demands both consistency and sincerity; one without the other won't do. We not only need to believe the other person will do the right thing, but will do it for the right reasons. Figure 1 summarizes the effects of high and low levels of consistency and sincerity on trust.

	HIGH CONSISTENCY	LOW CONSISTENCY
HIGH SINCERITY	High Trust	Mixed Message
LOW SINCERITY	Mixed Message	Low Trust

The condition of high consistency and high sincerity leads to trust, whereas the condition of low consistency and low sincerity leads to mistrust. The conditions of being consistent and insincere *("He's doing the right thing but doesn't really care about us")* and being inconsistent and sincere *("She cares about us but doesn't follow through")* send mixed messages that undermine trust.

Trust is such a crucial issue because we're aware that other people are capable of hurting us physically, emotionally, and financially. In other words, relationships with other people involve risk, and we're careful not to take risks unless we believe it's safe to do so. Our behavior will vary tremendously depending on whether or not we trust the other person. Some of these differences are depicted in Figure 2.

In the Trust Pattern, people are willing to make themselves vulnerable to another person because they believe it's safe to do so. In the Mistrust Pattern, however, people spend their time protecting themselves from a situation they perceive as threatening. When people are in this mode, often they react in ways that cause others to mistrust them, creating a vicious cycle.

Research by Dale Zand has shown that in teams where high-trust conditions exist, there is:

- more open discussion of ideas and feelings
- greater clarification of goals and problems
- a more thorough search for alternative courses of action
- a greater sense of influence by all participants
- more satisfaction with problem-solving efforts
- a greater desire to implement decisions
- a stronger feeling of team cohesiveness.

Results were the opposite in teams where low-trust conditions are present. Thus, it's very important to eliminate actions that lead to mistrust, and replace them with actions that build trust.

PATTERNS OF TRUST AND MISTRUST

Trust Pattern	Mistrust Pattern
Perception that the other person's behavior is consistent and sincere ↓ Conclusion that it's safe to trust ↓ Confidence ↓ Willingness to take risks	Perception that the other person's behavior is inconsistent and/or insincere ↓ Conclusion that it's not safe to trust ↓ Fear ↙ ↘ Fight (Attack to deal with perceived danger) — Flight (Escape or avoid perceived danger)

Actions Leading to Mistrust

A wide variety of actions can result in mistrust. Some of the more common examples are when team members:

- Say one thing but do another
- Make agreements they don't keep
- Say one thing to one person, something else to another
- Pretend to agree with others
- Try to discredit others
- Focus on other's mistakes
- Withhold information
- Make excuses for mistakes
- Undercut others
- Gossip about others
- Play politics to get what they want
- Form themselves into camps
- Seek win-lose outcomes
- Look out for their own interests
- Use manipulative tactics
- Make decisions affecting others without involving them
- Put each other down
- Blame others for mistakes
- Have hidden agendas
- Compete with each other
- Try to get even with each other
- Criticize each other
- Have a "we-they" mentality
- Openly attack each other
- Give more negative feedback than positive
- Spring surprises on others
- Ignore input from others
- Try to intimidate each other
- Use information to their own advantage
- Distort what people say.

Once trust has been violated, it's difficult to restore because people erect psychological barriers around their relationship with each other to protect themselves from getting hurt. Mistrust will continue indefinitely and become part of the corporate culture unless people are willing to confront trust issues directly, eliminate actions contributing to mistrust and engage in actions that will foster trust.

Suggestions for Enhancing Team Trust

Trust can be increased by replacing the negative actions discussed above with more positive actions. Some examples of such actions are as follows:

- Listen and convey understanding.
- Follow through on agreements.
- Resolve disagreements directly and in good faith.
- Say what you mean, mean what you say.
- Seek win-win outcomes.
- Be consistent in what you say to different people.
- Honor confidential information.
- Give others credit when it's due.
- Share information openly.
- Take responsibility for mistakes.
- Involve others in decisions affecting them.
- Avoid actions contributing to mistrust (gossip, blaming, etc.).
- Act out of integrity and not expediency.

Steps taken by teams to improve trust will help them become more successful because energy currently being wasted fighting each other can be redirected toward fighting the competition.

APPENDIX

3

Medical Office Business Processes

Accounts Receivable Management

- The obtainment of appropriate treatment authorizations and verification of insurance coverage
- Data entry (diagnoses, services, patient charges and contractual adjustments)
- Insurance billing (generation and sending of forms, or transmittal on-line)
- Patient billing (invoice entries and generation of bills)
- Logging payments on ledgers and depositing money in the bank
- Follow-up collections with insurance companies and patients
- Keeping current with billing codes and changes in reimbursement methods

Appointment Management

- New patient scheduling
- Follow-up visit scheduling
- Procedure scheduling

Medical Reporting

- Charting (writing in, filing, transporting and storing charts)
- Letters and reports to referring doctors
- Reports to third-party payers

Human Resource Development

- Employee job descriptions (empowerment)
- Employee training and education procedures (cross-training)
- Payroll, benefits and legal issues regarding personnel

Financial Management

- Accounts payable management (working capital and cash-flow management)
- Accounting procedures and budgeting
- Insurance needs
- Capital investment (e.g., lease or buy equipment; cost versus benefit analysis)
- Pension fund management (payroll and employee benefits)
- Managed care contract analysis (risk analysis)
- Capital structure (debt-versus-equity)

Inventory Management

- Medical supplies
- Custom supply storage and dispensing
- Office supplies and stationery
- Computer supplies

Patient Flow Management

- Room clean-up and set-up
- Patient movement from reception room to treatment room
- Patient movement to x-ray
- Patient movement from treatment room to front office and exit

Medical Procedures

- Instrumentation set-up for procedures
- Instrument sterilization and packaging
- Chairside assistance

General Management and Supervision

- Front office (business management)
- Back office (patient care management)
- Long-range strategic planning (downsizing and mergers)

NOTES